The Institute of Biology's
Studies in Biology no. 167

Blood-sucking Insects:
Vectors of Disease

Michael W. Service
D.Sc., F.I. Biol.

Reader in Medical Entomology,
Liverpool School of Tropical Medicine

Edward Arnold

© Michael W. Service, 1986

First published in Great Britain 1986 by
Edward Arnold (Publishers) Ltd, 41 Bedford Square, London WC1B 3DQ

Edward Arnold (Australia) Pty Ltd, 80 Waverley Road, Caulfield East.
Victoria 3145, Australia

Edward Arnold, 3 East Read Street, Baltimore, Maryland 21201, USA

British Library Cataloguing in Publication Data

Service, Michael W.
  Blood-sucking insects: vectors of disease.—
  (The Institute of Biology's studies in biology,
  ISSN 0537-9024; no. 167)
  1. Insects as carriers of disease   2. Bloodsucking animals
  I. Title   II. Series
  614.4'32   RA639.5

  ISBN 0-7131-2930-1

Text set in 9½/11 pt English Times Compugraphic
by Colset Pte. Ltd., Singapore.
Printed and bound by Camelot Press Ltd, Southampton.

General Preface to the Series

Because it is no longer possible for one textbook to cover the whole field of biology while remaining sufficiently up to date, the Institute of Biology proposed this series so that teachers and students can learn about significant developments. The enthusiastic acceptance of 'Studies in Biology' shows that the books are providing authoritative views of biological topics.

The features of the series include the attention given to methods, the selected list of books for further reading and, wherever possible, suggestions for practical work.

Readers' comments will be welcomed by the Institute.

1985
Institute of Biology
20 Queensberry Place
London SW7 2DZ

Preface

It is well to remember that blood-sucking insects are not exclusively a tropical problem. Admittedly it is mainly in the tropics that they are vectors of some of the worst scourges of mankind, such as malaria, sleeping sickness and river blindness, but it is very difficult to think of any country not having biting insects. In fact some biting flies, like mosquitoes, can be more numerous and troublesome in the cold subarctic regions than in the hot humid tropics.

Although we have amassed a powerful armoury of weapons to attack vector-borne diseases, we still have not yet won the war against them. In subsaharan Africa, for example, malaria is as rampant today as it was at the beginning of this century. It is a sobering thought that there are now more people infected with lymphatic filariasis than there were over a hundred years ago when Patrick Manson identified mosquitoes as the vector.

In discussing the various blood-sucking insects I have kept their morphological descriptions to a minimum to allow more space to describe their natural histories and the roles they play in disease transmission. I have also tried, albeit briefly, to outline the main clinical symptoms of the diseases spread by insects, and to indicate whether they can be prevented by immunization or prophylactic drugs or, once contracted, are curable. Any account of vector control rapidly becomes outdated, but because the principal strategy of disease control is so frequently based on killing the vectors, I have summarized the more important control methods.

Finally, emphasis has been directed at insects that bite and transmit disease to man, but where space has permitted I have also referred to veterinary pests and infections.

Liverpool 1985
M.W.S.

Contents

1 Biting Insects as Pests and Disease Vectors

1.1 Biting nuisances

In temperate as well as tropical countries blood-sucking insects can be so troublesome to man as to make life uncomfortable and in extreme cases unbearable. In Britain, for instance, although mosquitoes do not spread disease to man (in the past they transmitted malaria), they can be very annoying during the summer. Similarly, in the Camargue area of France, in Florida and California, mosquitoes can constitute a severe biting nuisance. In the subarctic and arctic regions of North America and Europe mosquitoes, together with simuliid blackflies, are so numerous as to make outdoor activities at certain times of the year difficult, if not impossible, unless protective clothing is worn. Very small biting midges (*Culicoides*) pestering visitors to the Scottish highlands led the Scottish Tourist Board during the 1950s to finance research into their biology and control. High densities of biting flies attacking cattle can also reduce milk yields and prevent weight gain.

For reasons still not fully understood, people differ in their attractiveness to mosquitoes and other biting flies, and also in their allergic responses to their bites. A person rarely bitten but showing severe allergic reactions may complain more about mosquitoes than someone who receives more bites but experiences little discomfort.

Despite simple and efficient control methods, obnoxious pests like bedbugs are still found in houses, though admittedly in many countries they are much less common than previously. Head lice are still commonly encountered in school children and are the bane of school staff.

1.2 Disease vectors

However troublesome insect bites may be, it is as disease vectors that they have gained notoriety. The Scottish physician Patrick Manson, working in China in 1878, was the first to find that insects could transmit disease to people – he identified mosquitoes as vectors of bancroftian filariasis. This discovery was some 20 years before two celebrated pioneers of medical parasitology, Giovanni Grassi in Italy and Ronald Ross in India, concluded that mosquitoes carried malaria. Although we can shuttle to the moon, we have failed in the more mundane task of conquering most insect-borne diseases. For example, while malaria has been eradicated from some areas it remains rife in most of the tropics (Fig. 1-1). Despite an excellent vaccine, yellow fever still flares up; in Ghana, for instance, there were 494 reported cases and 120 deaths in 1979 and 372 cases and 201 deaths in 1983. Another mosquito-borne disease, dengue, is invading new areas and has developed a more lethal form.

Some diseases such as plague, typhus and *falciparum* malaria quickly kill patients if they are not treated, but others like South American trypanosomiasis (Chagas' disease) run a chronic course of infection with death occurring only after many years. Other diseases are debilitating, such as river blindness (onchocerciasis) which as its name infers, causes loss of sight. Some infections produce unsightly deformities, like the grossly swollen limbs caused by lymphatic filariasis or facial disfigurations due to dermal leishmaniasis. Although tsetse flies transmit sleeping sickness and several thousand people may die annually, it is as vectors of cattle trypanosomiasis (nagana) that they are mostly studied, because this disease hinders agricultural and economic development in much of tropical Africa.

1.3   Methods of disease transmission

Parasitic infections are acquired and transmitted by insects in several different ways, some of which are remarkably simple but rather inefficient, while others are complicated and highly efficient. Some parasites can be transmitted by only a few species or just certain populations of a single species, while other infections are spread by several similar or very different species. Some of the basic principles of transmission are outlined below.

1.3.1   Mechanical transmission

This is the simplest form, there being neither multiplication nor cyclical development of the parasites in the vector; generally such infections can be spread by several different vectors. Myxomatosis is a good example. When mosquitoes, fleas and other biting insects feed on diseased rabbits, their mouthparts become contaminated with myxoma virus which is then readily transferred to healthy animals when they feed on them. The virus can remain dry and viable on the insects' mouthparts for many months. This method has been likened to insects being an infective 'flying pin'. Horseflies (tabanids) are mechanical vectors of *Trypanosoma evansi* to horses and camels, and while African trypanosomes are spread cyclically by tsetse flies, tabanids occasionally transmit the parasites through contaminated mouthparts. In these cases transfer of trypanosomes from one host to another must be within minutes because they cannot survive desiccation on the vector's proboscis. Interrupted feeding increases the chances of mechanical transmission because several hosts get bitten before the insect has obtained a full blood-meal.

1.3.2   Cyclical transmission

This describes the process by which parasites undergo multiplication and/or developmental changes within the vector. This necessitates an incubation period in the vector of a few days to a week or so to enable the

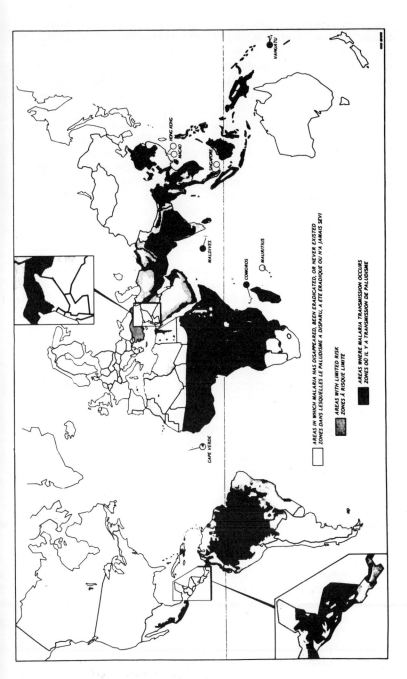

Fig. 1-1 The epidemiological status of malaria in 1981. (Courtesy of WHO.)

parasites to be in the 'correct' (infective) form in the right place (e.g. salivary glands, proboscis, faeces). Long-lived insects are therefore potentially better vectors of cyclically transmitted organisms than short-lived ones. A simple example of cyclical transmission is provided by typhus rickettsiae, which multiply in the gut cells of body lice before being excreted. If infected louse faeces are inhaled or rubbed into scratches or mucous membrances new infections arise. The rat flea is more efficient in transmitting plague bacilli, because, after they have multiplied in the flea's stomach, they are regurgitated into a host when the flea again tries to feed. After triatomine bugs have ingested trypanosome-infested blood from Chagas' victims, the parasites not only multiply in the bug's stomach but have to change into different morphological forms before infective parasites are produced in the faeces.

Not all parasites multiply in their vectors. For example, when the microfilariae of nematode worms responsible for river blindness and elephantiasis are ingested with a blood-meal many are destroyed in the gut of the vector, or are excreted. Only a few survivors migrate to the thoracic flight muscles, change into different morphological forms and pass to the proboscis. From here one or two infective larvae are deposited on a person's skin when the vector feeds; frequently they die but occasionally they manage to enter the vector's bite wound and establish a new infection.

Before sucking blood, most insects inject saliva into their hosts to prevent blood clotting in their delicate mouthparts. Consequently, parasitic development which involves the vector's salivary glands becoming infected is very efficient, as the parasites will be inoculated directly into a host and not just deposited on the skin. A simple example concerns viruses like yellow fever and dengue – which are known as arboviruses because they are *ar*thropod-*bo*rne *viruses*. After being taken up by a mosquito, the viruses multiply enormously and invade the salivary gland, from where they get pumped into subsequent hosts. Some protozoa, such as the trypanosomes causing African sleeping sickness, are also transmitted through saliva, but in this case not until they have completed a complicated migration through the tsetse fly's alimentary canal and proboscis.

The most sophisticated transmission cycle is that of malaria parasites, because not only do they multiply and migrate in the mosquito but also fertilization of gametes and formation of the zygote occurs in the vector. Eventually sporozoites are formed which invade the salivary glands.

1.3.3 Transovarial transmission

Viruses, spirochaetes and rickettsiae, in addition to being transmitted directly by the vector, occasionally penetrate their ovaries. As a consequence, young stages which hatch from eggs are already infected, and if they are blood-sucking, they can transmit the organisms to new hosts. Consequently each nymphal stage, and finally the adults, can transmit infections picked up by their mothers. Such hereditary transmission may persist for several generations before dying out. Transovarial transmission is most common in ticks and mites; in insects it is rarer, but the virus causing sandfly fever is transmitted transovarially by phlebotomine sandflies. More recently it has been discovered that a few arboviruses, including yellow fever, can pass transovarially through mosquitoes, but the mechanism does not appear to be very efficient.

1.4   Vector susceptibility

Parasites causing African trypanosomiasis can complete their development in any species of tsetse fly (all belonging to the genus *Glossina*), but only those species which commonly bite man are vectors of sleeping sickness. Similarly it seems that all American triatomine bugs (belonging to several genera) are capable of transmitting South American trypanosomiasis, but only those living in close association with man are actual vectors. In contrast to this lack of specificity, many other parasites will develop in only a few species within a genus. For example, human malaria develops in just a few of the many *Anopheles* species, and furthermore an *Anopheles* which transmits malaria in one region *may* sometimes be refractory to the same malaria parasites originating from a different area. In East Africa the mosquito *Culex quinquefasciatus* is an efficient host of bancroftian filariasis, whereas in West Africa it is not. Differences in susceptibility to parasites between species, and also between populations of the same species, are due to a variety of morphological and physiological factors which may limit or prevent the development of the parasites in the insects.

1.5   Zoonoses

Many diseases are zoonotic, that is they infect animals as well as man. Vector-borne examples include plague in rats, yellow fever in monkeys, Rhodesian type sleeping sickness in game animals, trypanosomes causing Chagas' disease in opossums, armadillos etc., and many forms of leishmaniasis parasites in rodents, dogs and other mammals. In many instances these wild animals provide important reservoirs of infection which can be passed on to man. The most effective reservoirs are those which do not die from the infection, but maintain it over long periods thus increasing the chance of disease transmission.

1.6   Prospects for disease control

A few diseases can be prevented by taking prophylactic drugs – malaria being the best known – or by vaccination (e.g. yellow fever), while others like typhus, plague and also malaria can be cured by chemotherapy. However, diseases such as river blindness, sleeping sickness and leishmaniasis are difficult to treat, and the drugs are often too toxic for mass administration in control campaigns. Because of such difficulties and problems of widescale drug distribution and drug resistance, resources have been concentrated on destroying the vectors. For example, malaria control is mainly based on spraying houses with residual insecticides to kill indoor-resting *Anopheles* mosquitoes, while rivers are dosed with insecticides to kill larvae of simuliid vectors of river blindness, and vegetation is sprayed to destroy the tsetse fly vectors of trypanosomiasis.

Although such control strategies have sometimes been successful, they have frequently failed, due partly to economic problems, inefficient spraying, changes in the behaviour of vectors allowing them to avoid sprayed surfaces, and insecticide resistance. Unfortunately insecticides have not been the panacea that was expected.

Eradication of most vector-borne diseases has to remain a 'pipe-dream'. At best the realistic goal must be to reduce transmission to an acceptable level, that is to a point where the disease is no longer a major public health problem. It seems that this will most likely be achieved by the combined use of insecticides, drugs, improved sanitation and housing, and health education. The adoption of such an integrated approach is, however, likely to prove difficult and time consuming.

Some of the more common or important diseases transmitted to humans by blood-sucking insects are summarized in the appendix.

2 Mosquitoes

To the general public mosquitoes are the best known of all biting insects, and they are probably the best studied of all economically important arthropods. There are more than 3100 species in 34 genera arranged in the three subfamilies – Toxorhynchitinae, Anophelinae and Culicinae – which comprise the family Culicidae. Mosquitoes have a worldwide distribution, breeding in the high arctic tundra as well as in dense tropical rain forests, but they are absent from Antarctica. Mosquitoes are pests in many areas, but their main importance is as vectors of diseases such as malaria, filariasis and yellow fever. Medically, the most important genera are *Anopheles, Culex, Aedes, Mansonia* and in Latin America also *Haemagogus*.

2.1 General biology

Adults are distinguished from other similar looking flies by having a long proboscis directed forwards, scales on the wing veins, a fringe of scales along the posterior border of the wing and head, and appressed scales covering the head, thorax, legs and abdomen. These scales are usually brown, black or whitish, but occasionally they are beautifully coloured and metallic-looking. Males are easily distinguished by their plumose antennae and by the length and shape of their palps (see Fig. 2-2).

Both sexes drink sugary secretions (e.g. nectar, honey) and females of most species, except those of subfamily Toxorhynchitinae, also suck blood from vertebrates (Fig. 2-1). Hosts range from the warm blooded mammals and birds to reptiles, amphibians and even, surprisingly, fish such as mudskippers and others that may lie partially out of the water. Species which bite man are termed anthropophilic while those feeding on other animals are often collectively called zoophilic, but bird-feeding species are sometimes distinguished as ornithophilic. These categories are rarely absolute, but rather describe feeding preferences. Some important disease vectors enter houses to feed on the occupants and are termed endophagic, but most mosquitoes prefer to bite out of doors (exophagic).

Host-seeking females are guided to their hosts mainly by body odours and carbon dioxide, but in some species visual stimuli, especially movements, are important. Most mosquitoes need at least one blood-meal before the ovaries can develop, that is blood is a requisite prelude to oviposition. These are known as anautogenous species to distinguish them from the few autogenous species which mature their first batch of eggs without taking blood, although blood is nearly always needed for subsequent ovipositions. Arctic mosquitoes may fail to find hosts and popula-

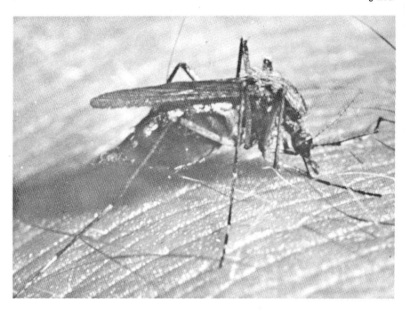

Fig. 2-1 A female *Aedes* mosquito completing her blood-meal. (M.W. Service.)

tions may survive for several generations by autogenous development, although they will readily feed on reindeer or other suitable hosts if they become available. Many mosquitoes bite only late at night while others are crepuscular; several species bite during the daytime and a few readily attack their hosts more or less throughout the 24-hour day. The behaviour of both mosquitoes and people can be relevant to disease transmission. For instance, disease vectors breeding and biting in forests will clearly attack only people entering forests, consequently hunters and wood cutters are more likely to become infected than those not visiting forests (see p. 21). A vector feeding early in the evening, out of doors in a village or town, is able to infect all members of the community, whereas an exophagic species active late at night will miss biting young children because they have gone indoors to bed.

Having fed, female mosquitoes seek suitable places in which to rest for a few days to allow their blood-meal to be digested and the ovaries to mature. Most mosquitoes rest out of doors (exophilic) in such places as amongst vegetation, in rodent holes and in cracks and crevices in the ground, but a few shelter in houses and are called endophilic. Exophily (outdoor resting) may have important implications in mosquito control (see p. 26). A question that is commonly asked, but one that is not easy to answer, is – how far do mosquitoes fly? It seems that frequently mosquitoes fly only a few hundred metres or so from their breeding places, although occasional flights of 1–2 kilometres are not unusual. There are also a few

well-documented reports of mosquitoes being blown several hundred kilometres by the wind, and sometimes such dispersal has lead to localised outbreaks of mosquito-borne diseases. The question of how long mosquitoes
live is also not easy to answer. In the tropics females probably live on
average 2–3 weeks, but many will die before this. In temperate regions they
often live for 6–8 weeks or longer, and some remain alive for many months
as fertilized and hibernating females. A very common temperate mosquito
which hibernates in cellars, outbuildings, sheds and the like, from about
September to April is *Culex pipiens*. Over most of its range it is not a pest of
man as it feeds exclusively on birds.

The immature stages of all mosquitoes are aquatic. Almost any type of
water can be a breeding place, but mosquitoes are absent from fast-flowing
waters and usually from lakes except amongst marginal vegetation. Larvae
are commonly found in swamps and marshes, ponds, pools, rainwater
puddles, rock pools, ricefields, ditches and drains. Some species thrive in
water highly contaminated with organic pollution such as in latrines, septic
tanks and other foul-smelling waters. A few species breed in saltwater
pools, marshes and tropical mangrove swamps. Usually such mosquitoes
are coastal, but they sometimes utilize inland saline waters, for instance in
Britain *Aedes detritus* breeds in the effluent of salt factories in Cheshire.
Several mosquitoes breed in man-made containers, like rainwater barrels,
cisterns, wells, water-storage pots, discarded tin cans, bottles and motor-
vehicle tyres. Others occur in natural container-habitats, such as rain-filled
tree holes (especially common in Europe in beech and sycamore trees), cut
bamboo stumps, water collecting in empty snail shells, split coconut husks,
and in the small amounts of water that accumulate in the leaf axils of
banana plants, pineapples and other plants. One of the more remarkable
breeding places is the water-filled pitcher of pitcher plants, which although
most numerous in south-east Asia also occur in North America, in fact
mosquitoes breed in pitcher plants growing not far from New York. Some
mosquitoes such as *Anopheles gambiae* can colonize a rather wide range of
habitats, such as ricefields, ponds, pools and puddles whereas others are
more or less restricted to a single type of habitat, such as *Aedes simpsoni*
which occurs in leaf-axils.

Despite mosquito larvae being aquatic, eggs are not always laid directly
on the water surface, for example *Aedes* species usually oviposit on wet
mud, leaf litter or other debris that subsequently becomes flooded. In
tropical countries eggs hatch within 2–4 days following oviposition but not
until 1–2 weeks in cooler temperate areas, and in some mosquitoes, such as
Aedes species, eggs may remain unhatched for months or even years.

Mosquito larvae can be distinguished from most other legless aquatic
insects by having a distinct head capsule bearing conspicuous feeding
brushes, followed by a bulbous thorax and a segmented abdomen with
numerous simple and branched hairs. The spiracles open on the last
abdominal segment, sometimes (e.g. in culicines) occurring at the end of a
siphon. Mosquito larvae regularly swim to the water surface to breathe in

air, except for those of *Mansonia* species which obtain their oxygen require-
ments from aquatic plants (see p. 13). Many larvae are filter feeders, others
browse and graze over bottom debris, while a few mosquitoes have predacious larvae which sometimes become cannibalistic. There are 4 larval
instars. In hot weather some tropical species complete larval development
within 4–5 days, but more usually the larval period lasts 10–12 days. In
temperate areas mosquitoes may remain as larvae for several weeks or
months, and a number of species overwinter as larvae.

The pupa has a segmented abdomen (terminating in a pair of paddle-like
structures) which, being curved underneath the cephalothorax, gives the
pupa a comma-shaped appearance. Pupae do not feed and spend most of
their time at the water surface breathing in air through the paired
respiratory trumpets situated on the cephalothorax. When disturbed they
dive in a rapid jerky manner. Pupae of *Mansonia* differ in that they remain
submerged with their respiratory trumpets inserted into plants (see p. 13).
Mosquitoes are one of the few groups of insects that have very mobile
pupae. In tropical conditions pupal life is only 2–3 days, but in temperate
areas it is often 10 days or so.

2.2 Classification of mosquitoes

Of the three subfamilies of the Culicidae, only the Anophelinae
and Culicinae contain disease vectors. In the third subfamily, the
Toxorhynchitinae (which contains a single genus, *Toxorhynchites*) the
proboscis is curved under the body and neither males nor females can bite.
Toxorhynchites is essentially tropical in its distribution (it is absent from
Europe but is represented in the USA and Canada). Adults are the largest of
all mosquitoes, some being 18 mm long. They have beautiful blue, green
and reddish iridescent body scales and black, white, red or yellow
abdominal hair tufts. Larvae occur mainly in tree-holes and are voracious
predators, and have occasionally been introduced into areas as biological
control agents, but usually with little success.

The following notes together with Figure 2-2 give the important differences between anopheline and culicine mosquitoes.

2.2.1 Anopheline mosquitoes

This subfamily contains three genera but only certain *Anopheles*, of
which there are more than 400 species, are disease vectors. *Anopheles*
species occur worldwide, being found in North America and Europe,
including Britain, as well as in tropical countries.

Adults usually rest at an angle to the surface (Fig. 2-2) and most have the
dark and pale scales on the wing veins arranged in 'blocks'. Male palps are
about as long as the proboscis and distinctly 'clubbed' apically; female
palps are equally long but are not swollen. Females mostly bite at night;
many species feed out of doors but some important malaria vectors bite and
rest in houses (i.e. are endophagic and endophilic). Eggs are laid on the

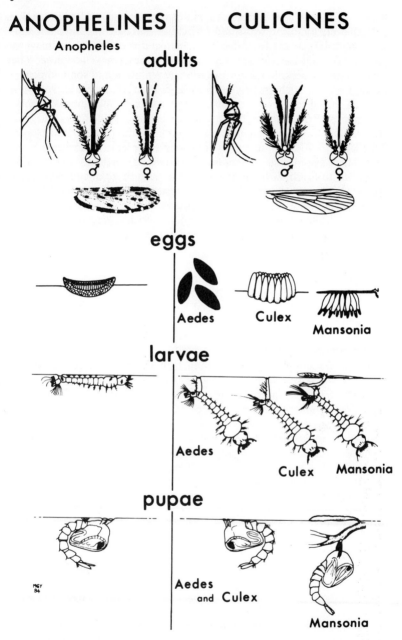

Fig. 2-2 Diagrammatic presentation of the principal differences between anopheline and culicine mosquitoes. (M.G. Yates.)

water surface and usually possess a pair of lateral air sacs called floats (Fig. 2-2); they are unable to withstand desiccation and hatch within a few days. *Anopheles* larvae are filter feeders and spend most of their time lying parallel to the water surface (Fig. 2-2). They never have a siphon. They favour clean waters, but a few can tolerate pollution and some important malaria vectors, such as *Anopheles melas* in West Africa and *A. sundaicus* in India, breed in saltwater habitats. A few species, including *Anopheles plumbeus* in Britain and *A. barberi* in the USA, live in tree-holes. Larvae of *A. bellator*, an important malaria vector in some parts of the tropical Americas, are found in leaf axils of bromeliads, plants which superficially resemble pineapples but are epiphytes on trees. It is not very easy for non-specialists to distinguish anopheline pupae from those of culicines, but in *Anopheles* the pupal respiratory trumpets are short and conical (Fig. 2-2).

Anopheles mosquitoes are well known vectors of malaria, but they also transmit filarial parasites (*Wuchereria bancrofti* and *Brugia malayi*) and a few arboviruses such as O'nyong nyong in East Africa.

2.2.2   Culicine mosquitoes

Thirty genera are included in this subfamily; the most important medically are *Culex, Aedes* and *Mansonia* which have a worldwide distribution, and additionally in Central and South America, *Haemagogus*. This subfamily can be distinguished from the Anophelinae as follows.

Adults rest with the body more or less parallel to the surface (Fig. 2-2) and scales on the wing veins are usually uniformly brown or blackish, although occasionally there is an admixture of pale and dark scales. Male palps are about as long as the proboscis and are not swollen apically (Fig. 2-2). The female palps are usually much shorter than the proboscis and consequently may be difficult to see. Females bite at night or during the day, most species feed and rest out of doors (exophagic and exophilic), but a few enter houses to feed and rest. Eggs may be laid as an egg raft floating on the water, as a sticky mass glued to vegetation or singly on damp surfaces (Fig. 2-2); they never possess floats. Larvae always have a short or long siphon by which they hang at an angle from the water surface (Fig. 2-2). They may be filter feeders, bottom browsers or, rarely, predacious on other mosquito larvae. Culicine mosquitoes have colonized almost all types of aquatic habitats, ranging from cesspits and saltwater pools, to water-filled flower bracts and leaf axils. Pupae having rather long respiratory trumpets can fairly easily be distinguished from anopheline pupae (Fig. 2-2), but those with short trumpets require microscopic examination for identification.

Culicine mosquitoes transmit filariasis, yellow fever, dengue and many other arboviruses, but not human malaria. They are also vectors of filarial worms and viruses amongst animals, and transmit avian malaria.

Culex   The genus has a worldwide distribution; adults are often brownish and lack conspicuous ornamentation. Eggs are unable to withstand desiccation and are usually deposited in an egg raft that floats on the water. Larvae, which have a short or long siphon with several pairs of subventral tufts, are commonly found in ground collections of water, including marshes, ponds, ditches and puddles. Adults mostly bite at night. *Culex pipiens* is a very common temperate species that is ornithophilic in most regions and overwinters as fertilized hibernating females. The closely related tropical *C. quinquefasciatus* (*fatigans*) breeds in septic tanks and other polluted waters; it is an important vector of bancroftian filariasis. *C. tritaeniorhynchus* transmits Japanese encephalitis in south-east Asia and its larvae are very common in ricefields.

Aedes Species of this genus are found worldwide, and in northern temperate areas they can be vicious biters. Adults are generally blackish, often with contrasting white or silvery markings on the body and legs. Eggs are laid singly on wet surfaces just above the water line, for example on damp mud and leaf litter, wet interior surfaces of tree-holes and clay pots; here they can resist drying out for many months and sometimes several years. Although ground collections of water often constitute breeding places, *Aedes* species have specialized in colonizing man-made and natural container-type habitats such as tin cans, pots, abandoned tyres, tree-holes, bamboo sections, leaf axils and rock pools. When eggs are immersed in water, frequently only a few hatch, subsequent immersions being needed to stimulate further hatching. Clearly an ability to withstand desiccation and hatch in instalments is advantageous for mosquitoes living in such temporary habitats. Larvae have short barrel-shaped siphons with only one pair of subventral tufts.

　　Aedes mosquitoes transmit several arboviruses, for example *A. aegypti* is a vector of yellow fever and dengue, *A. polynesiensis* helps spread bancroftian filariasis and *A. togoi* transmits brugian filariasis.

Mansonia These mosquitoes are essentially tropical, but a few species occur in temperate areas such as *Mansonia richiardii* in Europe, including Britain, and the closely related *M. perturbans* is common in the USA. Adults usually have the legs and body patterned with brown and whitish scales, while the wing veins are speckled with similar scales. Wing scales are broad and overlapping pairs give a heart-shaped appearance. Eggs are either deposited on the water as an egg raft, or glued as a sticky mass under-neath floating vegetation; they cannot withstand desiccation. Larvae have short conical siphons which are thrust into submerged parts of plants (e.g. *Salvinia, Eichhornia, Pistia*) so as to obtain oxygen from plant tissues. The pupal trumpets are also inserted into plants for respiratory purposes. Larvae and pupae remain attached to plants and rarely rise to the water surface. Obviously larval habitats must have vegetation; typically they comprise marshes, swamps, weedy ponds and ditches.

　　Adults are nocturnal and vicious biters. Some species transmit bancroftian and brugian filariasis.

Haemagogus   This genus is found only in Central and South America. Adults are small but highly coloured, having metallic green, blue and golden thoracic scales. Eggs can tolerate desiccation and are laid singly, mainly in tree-holes and bamboo stumps. *Haemagogus* larvae are similar to those of *Aedes*; differentiation is a task for specialists.

Adults bite in forests during the day, mostly high up in the tree canopy, but they sometimes descend to ground level. *H. falco* and other *Haemagogus* species are vectors of jungle yellow fever.

2.3   Medical importance

2.3.1   Biting nuisance

Many people think of mosquitoes as tropical insects, but they are troublesome pests worldwide, and are in fact often more numerous and annoying in northern temperate areas than anywhere in the tropics. Because of their long mouthparts they can bite through clothing unless it has a close weave. Reactions to the bites varies considerably amongst individuals (see p. 1); occasionally limbs become greatly swollen, while scratching can lead to secondary infections. Livestock sometimes suffer greatly from mosquitoes, and suffocation of young calves through inhalation of mosquitoes swarming round their heads has been recorded.

2.3.2   Malaria

Four species of parasites, namely *Plasmodium falciparum*, *P. vivax*, *P. malariae* and *P. ovale*, cause cases of human malaria. Malaria remains the most important tropical disease. It is variously estimated that 352 or 450 million people still live in highly malarious areas where there is no or little control of the disease (Fig. 1-1). In 1955 the World Health Organization considered that DDT and other residual insecticides would enable malaria to be eradicated, except from tropical Africa. Indeed malaria has been eradicated from Europe, the southern USA, northern Australia, Israel, Cyprus and a few small tropical islands, but alas not from the tropics. In 1969 the World Health Organization realized that eradication was unrealistic. They declared that the objective should be malaria control, that is, reducing malaria transmission to an 'acceptable level', or in other words reducing it to a point where malaria is no longer a major public health problem for a country. This still remains the general philosophy towards malaria. In some tropical countries there are, or have been, efficient malaria control programmes (in India malaria was reduced from about 75 million in 1947 to 0.1 million in 1965, but it rose again to about 10 million cases in 1977), whereas in other areas, such as subsaharan Africa, malaria is as widespread and common today as it ever was. Reasons for the lack of progress include the spread of insecticide resistance in the *Anopheles* vectors, and parasites becoming drug resistant. In many instances, however, malaria control has failed due to socioeconomic problems, such as lack of funds and trained manpower, breakdown of spraying procedures, poor surveillance, inefficient detection of malaria cases and general apathy.

Malaria formerly occurred in Britain, mainly in the counties of Essex, Cambridgeshire, Bedfordshire, Kent, Norfolk and Huntingdonshire, and was referred to as the ague (see Shakespeare's *Tempest* ii, 2; 68, 97, 139). Many famous people are reputed to have suffered from malaria, including Oliver Cromwell, James I, Charles II and Cardinal Wolsey. Malaria gradually declined and more or less died out in Britain during the 1890s due to a variety of reasons, including changes in farming and the life-style of rural people, and improved land drainage.

All malarias characteristically produce alternating chills and high fevers, the cycle of which lasts 3–4 days depending on the species of malarial parasite. The commonest two human malarias are caused by *Plasmodium falciparum* and *P. vivax*. The former is essentially tropical and subtropical and is the most lethal of all malarias, as reflected in its name, malignant tertian malaria, killing non-immune people within 1–2 weeks. It is the prevalent parasite in tropical Africa, probably causing one million infant deaths annually. Blackwater fever, which is now rare, refers to a condition caused by *P. falciparum* in which blood cells are broken down liberating haemoglobin into the plasma, which when excreted in the urine makes it blackish. This condition was aggravated by the irregular use of quinine. *P. falciparum* parasites can also cause the usually fatal cerebral malaria, in which brain capillaries become blocked with parasitized red cells. Fevers take on a 48 hour cycle and there are no relapses with *P. falciparum*. That is, there is no quiescent period followed a year or more later by new malaria attacks. By contrast *P. vivax* causes a milder disease (benign tertian malaria) which rarely results in death. It was formerly common in temperate regions, being responsible for malaria in Britain, but is now mainly confined to subtropical and tropical countries, being particularly common in the Indian subcontinent. Fevers occur at 48 hour intervals, and there are true relapses for up to 5 years, that is, the infection can remain dormant for several years followed by sudden new malarial fevers.

Life-cycle   The life-cycle of the malaria parasite is described in many text books (see Phillips (1983) for up to date account), and is therefore summarized only briefly here. Female *Anopheles* ingest male and female gametocytes with their blood-meal. Once in the vector's stomach, the male exflagellates and produces microgametes which fertilize female macrogametes. The resultant zygotes (ookinetes) penetrate the stomach wall and develop into oocysts, which rupture to produce thousands of sporozoites which migrate to the mosquitoe's salivary glands. Some 9–16 days after its infective blood-meal, the vector is infective and sporozoites are ready to be inoculated into a new host. Within an hour of inoculation, sporozoites have disappeared from the peripheral blood and have invaded the liver cells. Here they complete their pre-erythrocytic cycle of development, and after 7–10 days liberate merozoites, which invade the red blood cells and begin their erythrocytic cycle of development. Periodically gametocytes are produced; these are the only stages that can infect blood-feeding *Anopheles*. Some types of malaria (*P. vivax*, *P. ovale*) can maintain a reproductive cycle (exoerythrocytic cycle) in the liver, which can result in further releases of merozoites into the peripheral blood for up to 3 or even 5 years, giving rise to true relapses. Recent evidence suggests that in *P. vivax* and *P. malariae*, some sporozoites, called hypnozoites, may remain dormant in the liver for up to a year, before they start their pre-erythrocytic cycle in the liver, subsequently releasing merozoites into the blood system.

Immunity   The strongest immunity is that developed against *P. falciparum* and consequently is commonest in Africans. Children born to mothers infected with malaria are afforded some protection due to antibodies, mainly IgG, passing across the placenta, but this *passive* immunity disappears within 4–6 months. When infants are fed entirely on milk, their diet lacks para-amino benzoic acid, the absence of which seems to give additional protection against malaria, but possibly immune substances in breast milk also give some protection. If infants and children manage to survive repeated malaria infections and reach the age of 5–6 years, they will have developed considerable *acquired* immunity. Such persons are described as semi-immune; no one is totally immune to *P. falciparum* malaria. Immunity lasts only so long as people are regularly inoculated with parasites; if semi-immunes travel to non-malarious areas they lose their immunity after about 5 years, and on returning to Africa will suffer a few severe malaria attacks before regaining their immunity. This type of immunity can develop in all races and types of people, but some forms of immunity have a genetic basis, the best known being due to the aberrant sickle haemoglobin. Individuals heterozygous for sickle haemoglobin are referred to as showing sickle cell trait; about half their haemoglobin is normal (HbA) and half sickle haemoglobin (HbS). Now, although such people will readily become infected with malaria the number of parasitized erythrocytes (i.e. parasitaemia) is reduced, so the disease is less severe. Unfortunately those homozygous for HbS have 80% or more of their haemoglobin abnormal; they suffer from sickle cell anaemia and usually die before adolescence.

There are a few other genetic variants conferring some degree of immunity. For example, people deficient in the red-cell enzyme glucose-6-phosphate dehydrogenase (G-6-PD) appear to be afforded some protection against malaria. A high percentage of West Africans lack the Duffy antigen on their red cells and this gives good protection against *P. vivax*. British and American black people originating from West Africa have retained this genetic trait and are refractory to *P. vivax* malaria although they may not have been exposed to malaria for generations.

Treatment   There are several prophylactic drugs that, taken daily or weekly, give protection against malaria, so long as their use is continued for a month after leaving malarious areas. Some drugs give little protection against infection, but are effective in treatment, while others like chloroquine and quinine, serve as both prophylactic and curative drugs. A few drugs like the prophylactic paludrine inhibit the malaria cycle in the mosquitoes. Unfortunately resistance has developed to most antimalarial drugs. Resistance to chloroquine, one of the better curative drugs, was developed by *P. falciparum* during 1957 in Thailand, and is now prevalent in many other South American countries, in south-east Asia, parts of the Indian subcontinent and in 1978 reached East Africa. The menace of drug resistant strains of malaria is one of the curses of tropical medicine.

Vaccination   The search for an efficient vaccine is being vigorously pursued. The ideal would be a vaccine protecting against all species and strains of malaria, that is very long lasting and requires only one inoculation. This goal is unlikely to be attained for many years.

Malaria control   Malaria control in the past, and to a large extent even now, relies on killing the vectors with insecticide. This is done by either spraying larval habitats with organophosphate or carbamate insecticides, or applying residual insecticides like DDT, HCH or malathion to the interior surfaces of houses to kill indoor-resting adults (see mosquito control p. 26).

Vectors   Human malaria is transmitted by *Anopheles* mosquitoes, of which there are over 400 species, but only about 60 are important vectors. There are several features that determine whether or not an *Anopheles* carries malaria. Firstly, there must be no biochemical barriers to prevent the parasites completing their development within the mosquito; secondly, of course, the mosquito must bite people. *A. gambiae* is the principal vector in tropical Africa and is probably the world's most efficient one. This is because it has a marked preference for feeding on man, is long-lived, breeds prolifically in and around human habitations, and has a high infection rate of about 4–5%. In contrast, although *A. culicifacies* is the main vector in India, it frequently bites cattle in preference to man (thus reducing mosquito-man contact), has a lower survival rate, and an infection rate of 0.1% or less and consequently is not such a good vector.

Where efficient vectors breed prolifically throughout the year and temperatures allow transmission to be continuous, malaria becomes 'stable'. In such areas the adult population is semi-immune and is little affected by malaria, and this is the situation occurring throughout much of Africa. In India, Sri Lanka and many other areas, there are marked seasonal variations in vector densities and transmission becomes seasonal, with epidemics occurring in the monsoon period. Moreover, there may also be marked differences in malaria prevalences from year to year. In these situations malaria is described as 'unstable'; people have little chance of acquiring immunity, and as a result adults as well as children may suffer severely from malaria and die.

Frequently, man creats ideal breeding places for *Anopheles* vectors. For example, in the Indian subcontinent *A. stephensi* breeds in wells, water tanks, cisterns and other man-made structures commonly found in towns, and is responsible for most 'urban malaria'. In Sri Lanka, illegal gem miners who fail to fill in their pits after removing the precious stones create vast numbers of breeding places for *A. culicifacies*. Many malaria vectors, including *A. gambiae* and *A. culicifacies*, rapidly colonize irrigation schemes, particularly rice, so although such agricultural projects may increase food for the people they often also increase malaria transmission.

2.3.3 Filariasis

There are two important nematode worms transmitted to man that cause filariasis, namely *Wuchereria bancrofti* and *Brugia malayi*. Probably 400 million people are at risk of contracting mosquito-borne filariasis. The life-cycle of both species is similar. Engorging female mosquitoes ingest numerous microfilariae, many of which, however, are excreted by the vector or are destroyed in the gut. The few survivors pass across the stomach wall to the haemocoele and migrate to the thoracic flight muscles, where they become relatively inactive and turn into so-called 'sausage-shaped' forms. These moult twice to become 3rd stage infective larvae which pass through the head to rest in the fleshy labium of the mosquitoe's proboscis. The complete cycle takes 10 days or more. When the vector feeds again, one or two 3rd-stage larvae are deposited on the host's skin. Frequently they die, but occasionally they find an abrasion or bite wound, enter the host and invade the lymphatic system. After about a year, fertilized female adult worms liberate thousands of motile microfilariae which escape into the blood. Microfilariae live for about a year, and are produced continuously until the adult female worm dies, which may not be until 15–18 years have elapsed. After some time increasing damage to the lymphatic system and blockage of lymph nodes may result in limbs swelling (5–15% of cases), often to grotesque proportions (Fig. 2-3) and in the enlargement of the scrotum. This condition is known as elephantiasis.

Wuchereria bancrofti affects urban and rural communities in most tropical areas, from Latin America through Africa and Asia to the Pacific and extending into some subtropical regions. In most areas microfilariae exhibit marked nocturnal periodicity, being especially numerous in the peripheral blood between 2200 and 0100 hours, but very scanty or absent during the daytime, when they are in the blood vessels supplying the lungs. It follows that only night-biting mosquitoes can be infected, the most common vector being *Culex quinquefasciatus*, a mosquito that breeds in polluted waters of towns. Its vectorial capacity, however, varies; for example, while it is an efficient vector in East Africa it is a 'poor' one in West Africa, because the parasites mostly fail to develop in it. In rural areas *C. quinquefasciatus* is often of minor importance, transmission typically being maintained by *Anopheles* species; essentially any local

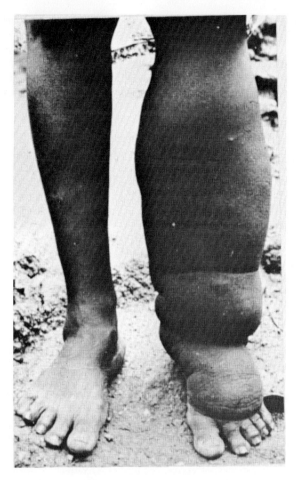

Fig. 2-3 Legs of a West Indian man suffering from elephantiasis caused by bancroftian filariasis. (Courtesy of M.B. Nathan.)

malaria vector is also a filarial vector.

Interestingly, microfilariae in people working at night show diurnal periodicity. A South Pacific strain of *W. bancrofti* is naturally diurnally periodic and is transmitted by day-biting *Aedes*, such as *A. polynesiensis* and *A. pseudoscutellaris*, but not *A. aegypti*. Man is the only vertebrate host, since bancroftian filariasis has no animal reservoir.

Brugia malayi is predominantly an infection of rural populations and has a much more restricted distribution, being found only in Asia, from India through south-east Asia to the south Pacific. It exists in two forms, the commonest of which is the nocturnal periodic form found from India to

Japan. The vectors are night-biting *Anopheles* and *Mansonia* mosquitoes. There are no animal reservoirs. The nocturnal form has a restricted distribution, but is found in Malaysia, Vietnam and the Philippines, and is essentially a disease of swamp-inhabiting monkeys. In addition to man, domestic and wild cats also become infected. This zoonotic filarial infection is spread by *Mansonia* species which bite during the day as well as at night.

Treatment The only drug used in mass chemotherapy is diethylcarbamazine (DEC) which, when given orally three times daily for 2–3 weeks, kills the microfilariae, and sometimes also the adult worms. Although DEC itself is relatively harmless, the toxic antigens released by thousands of killed microfilariae can cause nasty side-reactions such as fever, headache, vomiting and urticaria. Drugs that are more efficient at destroying adult worms are very toxic and have to be used with great caution, and cannot be administered routinely to populations. No drug can cure elephantiasis. Surgery can effectively rectify scrotal elephantiasis, but is unsatisfactory on enlarged limbs.

Filariasis control DEC has been administered in some areas, especially the Pacific, to reduce the reservoir of microfilariae in people, but insecticidal campaigns aimed at the vectors are a major control strategy in most areas.

2.3.4 Yellow fever

Yellow fever is caused by an arbovirus and is essentially a zoonotic disease of forest monkeys in Africa and Central and South America that sometimes spreads to man. In the past it occurred as far north as Baltimore and Philadelphia in the USA, and was brought by ship to Europe; there were minor yellow fever outbreaks in Swansea, Wales in 1865 and in Southampton, England in 1852. The disease cannot establish itself in Europe because the relevant vectors are absent. However, in Asia where the urban vector (*Aedes aegypti*) is exceedingly common and Indian *Macaca* monkeys are very susceptible to the virus, for some unexplained reason yellow fever has not become established.

After a person or monkey has become infected, the virus appears in the peripheral blood after an incubation period of only 3–6 days. However, such viraemia only lasts 3–4 days after which, if the host survives, it is immune for life and viraemia is never again produced. Therefore, a person or monkey is infective to mosquitoes for just 3–4 days. As with many other viral diseases, many people may become infected and show no obvious symptoms, but nevertheless they will have acquired life-long immunity. When clinical symptoms appear they include high fever, headache, pains in the limbs, black vomit and yellowing of the conjunctiva. Later the skin becomes yellowish, giving rise to the name of the disease. Overall mortality is 5–10%, but can be much higher, for example, it was estimated as about

85% in the 1960–62 Ethiopian epidemic. This was the last big epidemic killing at least 15 000, and possibly 30 000, people. Small outbreaks continually flare up in West Africa and South America, for example 109 cases were identified in Colombia in 1978 of which 20 people died, and in 1982 all 25 cases detected in the Ivory Coast, West Africa, died. In 1983 there were 728 cases, including 487 deaths in West Africa (see also p. 1).

When ingested by a mosquito, the virus passes through the stomach wall into the haemocoele and subsequently to the salivary glands where it multiplies. After 12–15 days, the mosquito becomes infective and the virus is inoculated along with saliva when it feeds. It has recently been discovered that yellow fever virus, at least in the laboratory, can be transovarially transmitted, but the extent to which this happens in wild populations of mosquitoes needs to be assessed.

In Africa, yellow fever virus infects cercopithecid monkeys inhabiting forests, but it has very little effect on them, and they rarely die. Monkey-to-monkey transmission is maintained by *Aedes africanus*, a forest mosquito that breeds in tree-holes and feeds mainly at around sunset in the tree canopy. This sylvatic or forest cycle maintains the reservoir of yellow fever in the monkey population (Fig. 2-4). Occasionally more adventurous monkeys raid farms at the edge of the forests and may get bitten by *A. simpsoni*, a species that breeds in water-filled leaf axils of bananas and pineapples, and which bites during the daytime. If monkeys are viraemic then *A. simpsoni* can spread the virus to other monkeys and to people; this is the rural cycle of transmission. When an infected person returns to his village or travels to town he is likely bitten by *A. aegypti*, a mosquito that colonizes water-storage pots, tin cans, abandoned tyres and other man-made containers. This mosquito is responsible for the urban cycle of transmission and yellow fever epidemics. A few other mosquitoes have been incriminated as vectors, but the three referred to here are undoubtedly the most important vectors in Africa.

In Central and South America the epidemiology of yellow fever differs in certain respects. Again it is a disease of forest monkeys, mainly cebid ones, but they are more susceptible than African monkeys and often fall sick and die. In fact, the existence of jungle yellow fever is often first recognized by a trail of dead monkeys. Transmission amongst Central and South American monkeys is again by jungle-dwelling mosquitoes, that breed in tree-holes and bite high up in the forest canopy. The most important vectors are various *Haemagogus* species, especially *H. falco* and *H. leucocelaenus*, and to a lesser extent, *Sabethes chloropterus*. When wood cutters enter forests to fell large jungle trees, the canopy-inhabiting mosquitoes descend to bite them, and if they are infected then the workers contract yellow fever. This is the jungle or sylvatic cycle (Fig. 2-5). The urban cycle, as in Africa, is transmitted by the domestic *Aedes aegypti*. There is no rural cycle.

Vaccination   There is no specific treatment for yellow fever victims, so emphasis is on prevention. Vaccination gives protection for at least 10

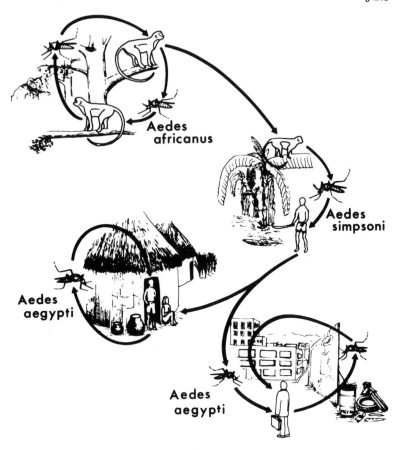

Fig. 2-4 Diagrammatic representation of the yellow fever cycles in Africa. (M.G. Yates.)

years, but not immunity for life as is usually achieved when a person survives a natural attack of yellow fever. This is because the vaccines are not as efficient as the wild virus. One of the more successful vaccines, named 17D, originated from Mr Asibi in Ghana in 1927 who contracted, and survived, a highly virulent strain of yellow fever. Control of yellow fever epidemics is based on vaccination and insecticidal campaigns against the urban vector *A. aegypti.*

2.3.5 Dengue

Aedes aegypti is the principal vector of dengue, an almost exclusively urban arboviral disease that occurs in 4, 5 or perhaps 6 different serological forms (e.g. dengue types 1,2,3, etc). Classical dengue is a relatively mild, non-fatal febrile disease producing a rash and pains in the joints, which is

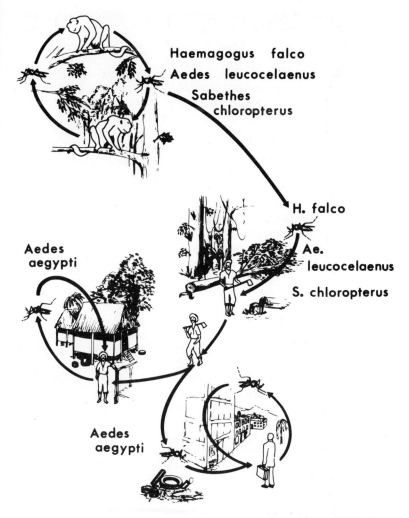

Fig. 2-5 Diagrammatic representation of the yellow fever cycles in Central and South America. (M.G. Yates.) The mosquito *A. leucocelaenus* has been transferred to the genus *Haemagogus*.

encountered in most tropical countries and sometimes in temperate regions. Dengue has been increasing in the Caribbean and epidemics now occur almost yearly. In 1954 a new form of dengue, termed haemorrhagic dengue, flared up in the Philippines, then spread to other south-east Asian countries, the western Pacific and more recently to the Caribbean area. This is a virulent disease most commonly found in children, characterized by bleeding in the skin and from the gums, nose and uterus, by internal haemorrhages, and shock. It has been responsible for killing a large number of children, and there is an overall mortality rate of about 10–20%. After yellow fever, this form of dengue has claimed more deaths than any other arboviral infection.

There are no significant animal reservoirs of either type of dengue, though it has been suspected that certain Malaysian monkeys may harbour the virus. There are no specific drugs to prevent or treat dengue. Control is aimed at killing the mosquito vectors (see page 26).

2.3.6   Encephalitis arboviruses

Many of the encephalitis viruses, so-called because they sometimes invade the central nervous system and brain, are mosquito-borne. Several are zoonoses, common in North America, with birds usually as reservoir hosts and man as the incidental one. In severe cases, patients suffer damage to the brain and motor nerves and symptoms rather like poliomyelitis develop; the death rate in the USA can be about 10%. Frequently, however, there is no or little involvement of the central nervous system and the most obvious manifestation is a fever and headache, while at other times infections are asymptomatic. Several of the encephalitis viruses infect horses, sometimes killing them, and are consequently known as equine encephalitis viruses. For example, Venezuelan equine encephalitis (VEE), which is found in southern USA, through Central America to northern South America, is transmitted mainly by *Culex* and *Aedes* mosquitoes and is greatly feared in the USA as it kills horses. Apart from man, horses, rodents and birds are important hosts. Eastern equine encephalitis (EEE) occurs mainly in eastern USA, but extends down to South America. *Culiseta melanura* transmits the virus amongst birds, while *Aedes* species spread it to horses and man. Western equine encephalitis (WEE) occurs in western and other parts of the USA down into parts of South America, and again is basically an infection of birds that also occurs in man and horses. The principal vector is *Culex tarsalis*, a very common ricefield-breeding mosquito. St Louis encephalitis (SLE) is reported widely in the USA and extends to South America; it is spread by *C. quinquefasciatus* and other *Culex* mosquitoes. In addition to infecting wild birds, in towns it is found in poultry.

An important non-American virus is Japanese encephalitis (JE) which occurs from India through south-east Asia to Japan. The basic transmission cycle involves birds such as herons, egrets and ibises, but pigs are also important reservoirs because they develop high viraemias and thus provide a ready source of infection to mosquitoes; they consequently act as amplifying hosts. Transmission to birds, pigs and man is chiefly by *C. tritaeniorhynchus*, a mosquito that breeds prolifically in ricefields. Much pig-to-pig transmission seems to be by *C. gelidus*.

The viraemia produced in man by JE, EEE, VEE, SLE and sometimes by WEE is so low that mosquitoes cannot usually ingest sufficient virus for it to replicate in the vector and make it infective. Man is therefore regarded as a 'dead-end' host. Similarly, when horses are involved they are also 'dead-end' hosts.

Horses can be successfully vaccinated against Venezuelan equine encephalitis, and although vaccines have been produced for WEE and JE, SLE and even dengue, for various reasons they are not widely used. Prevention and control is based on insecticidal attack on the vectors.

2.3.7 Other arboviruses

Many other arboviruses are spread by mosquitoes, such as West Nile fever (Africa, Europe, Asia and Israel), Rift Valley fever (Africa), Chikungunya (Africa and Asia), Bunyamwere (Africa) and Murray Valley encephalitis (Australia and New Guinea). In Britain, mosquitoes do not transmit viruses to man, but in southern France, Italy and Czechoslovakia and other European countries *Aedes* species spread Tahyna virus.

It was originally considered that mosquito-borne viruses were transmitted only by culicine mosquitoes (mainly *Aedes* and *Culex*), but in 1959 an epidemic of a previously unrecognized virus occurred in Uganda, subsequently named O'nyong-nyong, which was transmitted by *Anopheles gambiae* and *A. funestus*, the two major African malaria vectors. Later O'nyong-nyong was discovered in other East African countries. At present about 22 other arboviruses have been isolated from *Anopheles* mosquitoes in different parts of the world.

2.3.8 Animal parasites

In addition to zoonotic diseases (e.g. many viral infections and subperiodic *Brugia malayi*) mosquitoes transmit several parasites to domestic and wild animals, but very few are of major economic importance.

Plasmodium knowlesi and *P. cynomogli* are malaria parasites of monkeys, while *P. berghei* is a common African rodent malaria; all three are transmitted by *Anopheles*. In contrast *P. gallinaceum* is transmitted by *Aedes* mosquitoes to chickens and other birds. Ronald Ross (Section 1.2) did much of his pioneering work in India on malaria transmission using *P. relictum* in sparrows.

Brugia pahangi is a south-east Asian filarial parasite transmitted by *Mansonia* mosquitoes to cats and wild carnivores in Malaysia. Several other filarial worms, for example, species of *Setaria*, are transmitted to ungulates, but cause no apparent harm. In North and South America, India, China, Japan, Australia and southern Europe, but not Britain, the filarial worm, *Dirofilaria immitis* causes a disease known as dog heartworm, which can be a major veterinary problem often causing death in pets. It is spread by both anopheline and culicine mosquitoes. There are several other filarial infections of wild and domesticated animals.

2.4 Mosquito control

Mosquito control is undertaken in most countries; even in Britain breeding places may be sprayed during the summer. Some of the best organized and most extensive control operations are practiced in the USA, where mosquitoes are not only a biting nuisance but vectors of encephalitis viruses to people and horses.

Control methods can be conveniently divided into three main divisions – insecticidal, physical and environmental, and biological.

2.4.1 Insecticidal control

In the past, mineral oils (e.g. diesel, kerosene) and Paris green dusts were regularly applied to aquatic habitats. The former killed not so much by suffocating larvae as by the release of toxic aromatic hydrocarbons, while Paris green (copper aceto-arsenite) acted as a stomach poison. Although resistance has not developed to these chemicals, they have more or less been abandoned in favour of organophosphate (e.g. malathion, chlorpyrifos, temephos, pirimiphos-methyl) and carbamate (e.g. carbaryl) insecticides which although admittedly killing non-target aquatic life, are at least biodegradable and hence do not accumulate in the environment.

In tropical countries, spraying has to be repeated about every 7–10 days, but less frequently in temperate regions. If very large or inaccessible areas are to be treated, aerial applications may be necessary. Herbicides like paraquat may be useful in ridding waters of *Mansonia* mosquitoes as their host plants are destroyed.

Insecticidal fogs and aerosols of malathion or synthetic pyrethroids, produced from vehicle-mounted machines or from aircraft, have proved very successful in combating epidemics of dengue, yellow fever and occasionally other diseases, as well as being generally effective in killing mosquitoes resting out of doors. Usually the effect is short-lived because treated areas are quickly reinvaded from untreated areas, or by newly emerged mosquitoes. Consequently repeated applications over several days or weeks may be necessary.

The application of $2\,\text{gm}^{-2}$ of DDT wettable powder to the interior surfaces of houses twice a year is very effective in killing endophilic malaria vectors, in fact most malaria control campaigns have been based on this strategy. If resistance appears, other insecticides like HCH (BHC) or malathion can be used, but they are more expensive and may have to be sprayed 3–4 times a year. Indoor spraying will also kill other house-resting mosquitoes, such as *Culex quinquefasciatus*, as well as certain phlebotomine sandflies (see p. 38) and triatomine bugs (see p. 70), but is clearly ineffective against exophilic vectors.

2.4.2 Physical and environmental methods

This category includes drainage of marshes, filling in ponds, and removing abandoned tin cans, tyres and other man-made habitats. In the tropics, repairing defective soak-way pits can greatly reduce breeding by *C. quinquefasciatus*. If water-storage pots have tight-fitting lids, or the water is changed weekly, this should exclude *A. aegypti*. Sometimes a habitat can be altered to make it unsuitable, for example by removing overhanging vegetation to eliminate shade-loving mosquitoes, but care is needed to ensure that such changes do not attract other species.

Sometimes, instead of being drained, wetlands are dug out to form ponds with well defined vertical banks. Such impoundments are unattractive to *Aedes* mosquitoes because there are no areas of wet mud suitable for egg laying, but other species, e.g. *Anopheles* and *Culex*, may find these new habitats ideal breeding places. Fish and ducks can be introduced to impoundments to make them more attractive and also to give some degree of biological control.

2.4.3 Biological control

Although biological control has had some notable successes against agriculturally important pests, it has been far less successful against mosquitoes and other medical vectors. With plant pests, the main aim is to reduce populations to a level where crop damage becomes acceptable, but with vectors, much greater reductions are usually needed to produce any significant decrease in disease transmission.

The best known biological control agent is the top minnow or 'mosquito fish' *Gambusia affinis*, a native of the southern USA which has been introduced into many tropical and subtropical countries to devour mosquito larvae. Another fish, the guppy *Poecilia (Lebistes) reticulata*, has the advantage of surviving better in organically polluted waters, but is not so voracious as *Gambusia*. Although fish undoubtedly reduce larval populations in specific breeding places, there is little convincing evidence that they substantially reduce either biting nuisances or disease transmission. Nevertheless, fish are used routinely in many countries, such as in ricefields in China, Japan and California, in wells and water cisterns in Indian towns, in anopheline larval habitats in Iran, and in mosquito-infested coconut-husk pits in Sri Lanka.

Amongst parasite-based control methods, one of the more successful is use of the nematode *Romanomermis culicivorax* against mosquito larvae, but it is not effective against all species. Moreover, it cannot develop in brackish or polluted habitats and even in freshwater frequently fails to survive and recycle, so necessitating repeated nematode applications. In the laboratory a few mosquitoes have developed resistance to nematodes, either by melanizing and encapsulating the parasites or somehow avoiding contact with them.

There are numerous viruses, bacteria, protozoa and fungi that parasitize mosquito larvae, and a few have shown some potential as biocontrol agents. The most promising is *Bacillus thuringiensis* var. *israelensis* (or serotype H–14), which also destroys larval simuliids (see p. 33). Mortality is caused by ingestion of endotoxins produced by bacterial spores. Commercial formulations of *B. thuringiensis* var. *israelensis* consist of dead bacteria and endotoxins; there is no survival or multiplication of the bacteria and breeding places have to be repeatedly sprayed. It is more of a microbial insecticide than a true biological control agent.

There are several genetical methods for insect control, one of the commoner being the sterile-male release approach. For this, the mosquito species in question must be mass reared and the adults sterilized, for example, by rearing larvae in water containing chemosterilants. Sterilized males are then released into wild populations in the hope that they inseminate a high proportion of newly emerged females before wild males do so. This will result in the production of sterile eggs. An experimental test of the method was undertaken in El Salvador, where the principal malaria vector, *Anopheles albimanus*, is resistant to many insecticides. In a trial over 5 months 4.36 million sterile males were released. This achieved a very large reduction (99.9%) in larval population, but only in a specially selected and isolated area of 14 km². Elsewhere, genetic control experiments with mosquitoes have generally been disappointing, often because of poor vigour and mating competitiveness of the sterilized males, dispersal of fertilized females from outside the experimental area, or logistic problems.

Although biological control methods may seem attractive, unfortunately they require better understanding of the population dynamics of the vectors than do other control methods. Moreover, as they are slow-acting, they are unsuitable in emergencies such as disease epidemics, where insecticides are more appropriate.

2.4.4 Personal protection

Houses and hospitals can be screened to exclude mosquitoes, but good maintenance is needed to prevent screening from deteriorating and becoming ineffective. Mosquito nets can also provide protection against those species that bite late at night. Both screening and nets make sleeping conditions hotter and in developing countries may be too costly for general use. In addition in many village-type houses nets take up too much space to be placed over all sleeping occupants.

Suitable repellents like dimethylphthalate (DMP) and diethyl toluamide (DET) can give some degree of protection, but their effect wears off after about 2 hours. However, if clothing is impregnated with repellents it may remain effective for several months.

3 Blackflies

Blackflies belong to the family Simuliidae and most species and certainly most disease vectors belong to the genus *Simulium*. Blackflies have a worldwide distribution and can be exceptionally numerous and troublesome in subarctic areas of Canada and Europe. It is in Africa, however, that they constitute the greatest potential health hazard, because here they are vectors of the debilitating disease, river blindness (onchocerciasis).

3.1 Biology of blackflies

Adults are rather small (1.5–4 mm), stout-bodied and usually blackish insects, though many species have silvery, golden or orangy hairs on the thorax and legs giving them a distinctly patterned appearance. The 11-segmented antennae are relatively short and without conspicuous hairs, they are often described as cigar-shaped. The mouthparts are short and hang down from the head (Fig. 3-1d). In females the eyes are distinctly separated (dichoptic), but in males they meet along the dorsal surface of the head (holoptic) (see also tabanids). The relatively large thorax is rather humped and bears a pair of colourless and membraneous broad wings, characteristically with only a few well developed veins.

The immature stages of blackflies live in running waters; larval habitats range from slowly flowing irrigation channels to large fast flowing rivers such as the Volta, Nile and Niger in Africa.

In many species, females partially submerge themselves in a stream to glue their ovoid eggs (Fig. 3-1a) onto submerged vegetation or stones in a sticky mass or chain. In other species eggs are dropped from females flying over streams and rivers. In tropical countries, the eggs hatch within 1–4 days, but in cooler temperate areas they may remain unhatched for several weeks, and a few species pass the winter as diapausing eggs. The larva has a dark head – this contrasts with its paler body which is usually, with few exceptions, swollen posteriorly. A diagnostic feature of the larva is the proleg, situated ventrally just behind the head and armed with a small circle of hooklets (Fig. 3-1b). Larvae do not swim, but remain attached to rocks and vegetation by another circle of hooks situated at the posterior end of the body. Using the proleg and posterior hooklets, larvae can progress in a looping fashion, reminiscent of some caterpillars. Alternatively, they can fix a droplet of sticky saliva to a suitable substrate and release their hold to drift downstream on a silken thread; they can then either find a new attachment site or swallow their thin 'anchor-line' and regain their original position. In a few species larvae and cocoons are attached to crustaceans,

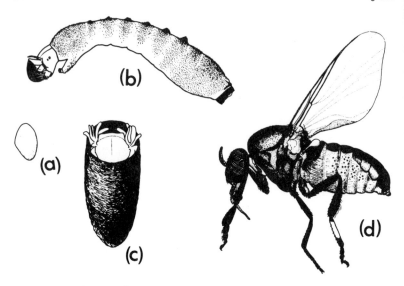

Fig. 3-1 *Simulium* species: (**a**) egg; (**b**) larva; (**c**) pupa in cocoon; (**d**) adult female. (Modified from Smith, 1973, courtesy British Museum (Nat. Hist.) London.)

the best known example being *Simulium neavei* of eastern Africa which is phoretic on *Potomonautes* crabs.

Blackfly larvae are filter feeders and the head bears a prominent pair of cephalic fans, often called mouthbrushes, which strain food particles from the water. There are 6–8 larval instars. In tropical countries, larval life is about 7–14 days, but in temperate regions many months may be spent as larvae and several species overwinter in this stage. The last larval instar – easily recognized because it has a black 'gill spot' on each side of the thorax – spins a silken slipper-shaped cocoon (Fig. 3-1c), which is firmly attached to submerged rocks or vegetation. The pupa, enclosed within its protective cocoon, bears anteriorly a conspicuous pair of branched filamentous or stoutish respiratory gills. Pupal duration, whether in temperate or tropical countries, is only about 2–6 days. Adults emerge under water and either crawl up vegetation to the surface or float up in a bubble of air. Once they have broken through the water surface they fly off.

Only female blackflies take blood-meals; males live on naturally occurring sugary secretions. In addition to man, adult females will bite cattle and numerous other mammals, while some species feed almost exclusively on birds. Biting is almost entirely restricted to the daylight hours and takes place out of doors; it tends to be most intense near streams and rivers. There are often preferred feeding sites, for instance in Africa *Simulium damnosum* bites people mostly on the legs, whereas *S. ochraceum* in South America feeds mainly on the upper parts of the body.

Several blackfly species are adept at entering the ears of animals to feed, while others concentrate on biting the belly of cows and similar hosts. Many species are capable of flying long distances. In Canada *S. arcticum* often flies several hundred kilometres, while the important vector of onchocerciasis in Africa, *S. damnosum*, can disperse on the prevailing winds up to 300 km, possible even 500 km, from its breeding places. Such dispersal can make vector control difficult.

3.2 Medical and veterinary importance

Blackfly bites can be painful and give rise to swellings. Some people suffer from dermatitis after prolonged exposure to being bitten. This is partly due to the rasping action of blackfly mouthparts during feeding, but also to antigenic reactions following the injection of saliva. In northern Canada, attacks at certain times of the year can be so serious as to virtually preclude outdoor activities. Hordes of blackflies biting cattle can reduce milk yields and beef production.

3.2.1 Onchocerciasis

Although simuliids can be troublesome pests, it is as vectors of onchocerciasis (aptly named river blindness because the vectors breed in rivers and the disease can result in people becoming blind) that they are most important. Onchocerciasis is found only in West, Central and East Africa between latitudes of about 15°N and 13°S, in small foci in southern Yemen and Saudi Arabia and a few restricted areas in Mexico, Guatemala, Equador, Venezuela, Colombia and Brazil. About 20 million people are currently infected with onchocerciasis. The worst foci occur in West Africa, especially in the Volta River Basin where some 10% of the population harbours the infection, and about 70 000 of the 10 million inhabitants are completely, or almost completely, blind.

The causative agent is the nematode worm *Onchocerca volvulus*, which is found in the subcutaneous tissues of man. Adult worms themselves, although living in people for as long as 15–18 years, do little harm, despite the fact that they may form nodules just under the skin. Trouble occurs only when thousands of minute microfilariae are liberated by female worms and invade the skin, including the eyes. The accumulation and death of large numbers of these minute filarial worms in the skin causes intense itching, a papular eruption, loss of elasticity leading to a wrinkled and pre-maturely-aged appearance, and sometimes depigmentation causing a condition known as 'leopard skin'. However, by far the worst pathological aspect of the disease is damage to the eyes, resulting in gradual deterioration of vision, and possibly total blindness (Fig. 3-2).

The rather blunt mouthparts of a female blackfly rasp the skin during feeding, liberating the skin-inhabiting microfilariae which are consequently taken up with the blood-meal. Many of the ingested microfilariae are killed within the fly or excreted, but a few survive, migrate across the stomach

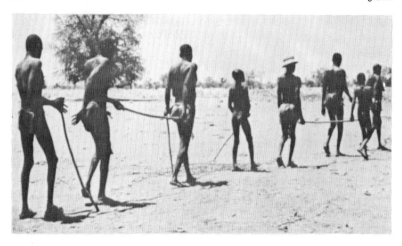

Fig. 3-2 A group of people in West Africa blinded by onchocerciasis being lead from a village. (Courtesy of WHO.)

wall into the haemocoele and from there invade the insect's thoracic flight muscles. Here they change firstly into sausage-shaped worms, then into longer and thinner individuals which pass through the head capsule down into the labium of the mouthparts. Depending on temperature, this cyclical development takes 6–14 days. When an infective fly bites a person one or two infective 3rd-stage worms are deposited on the skin. Frequently these worms die, but if they manage to enter the bite wound they infect man and after about 18 months, fertilized adult female worms start producing microfilariae.

The major vectors of onchocerciasis in Africa belong to the *Simulium damnosum* complex, which cytological studies on larval salivary glands have shown to comprise at least 26 distinct species; luckily not all are vectors. In Uganda and the two Congo Republics, *S. neavei*, the immature stages of which are phoretic on crabs, is a vector. In America the principal vectors are *S. ochraceum*, *S. metallicum*, *S. exiguum* and the *S. amazonicum* group.

Suramin can be used to kill adult worms in man, but there can be serious toxic effects, making it unsuitable for mass administration. Under close medical supervision, a very few drugs such as DEC (diethylcarbamazine) can be given to kill the microfilariae; even so patients are likely to suffer side-reactions such as intense itching, nausea, giddiness and very occasionally, death. Moreover, the beneficial effects of treatment are short-lived because unaffected female adult worms are continually releasing microfilariae into the skin. Because of the lack of a safe cure that can be administered on a wide scale, the only method for controlling the disease relies on killing the vectors (see Section 3.3).

3.2.2　Other diseases

In Brazil, and possibly elsewhere, *S. amazonicum* transmits to man *Mansonella ozzardi*, a filarial worm generally regarded as non-pathogenic (see also p. 41). The virus responsible for Venezuelan equine encephalitis can apparently be spread by simuliids as well as by the more normal mosquito vectors (p. 24).

Blackflies also transmit *Onchocerca gutturosa* and *O. linealis* to cattle in Britain, *O. ochengi* to cattle in Africa and various other filarial infections to wild and domesticated animals, including birds. Finally, protozoans of the genus *Leucocytozoon* are transmitted to both wild and domesticated birds, and can cause disease in ducks (*L. simondi*) and turkeys (*L. smithi*). For this reason, they are economically important in North America.

3.3　Control methods

Blackfly (and onchocerciasis) control is virtually restricted to applying insecticides to breeding places to kill the larvae. Originally organochlorines like DDT were used in Africa and North America, but because of their persistent residues they are no longer acceptable. Instead, organophosphates such as temephos (Abate) are employed. Insecticidal applications are made from bridges or the banks of rivers, or where appropriate from helicopters and fixed-wing aircraft. Treatment is usually repeated every 7–14 days, the interval depending on the rate of larval development; in cold climates much less frequent dosing may suffice.

In an ambitious Onchocerciasis Control Programme (OCP) organized by the World Health Organization in 1974, all blackfly breeding places in the Volta River Basin in West Africa were given weekly aerial dosing with temephos. The aim has been not so much to eradicate the vector as to reduce its numbers to the level where the transmission cycle is broken and eventually the parasite reservoir in man dies out, so that if areas are reinvaded by blackflies there will be no *Onchocerca* worms to be transmitted. The control area now covers about 764 000 km² and involves parts of Ghana, Mali, Niger, Burkina Faso (Upper Volta), Togo, Benin, and the Ivory Coast. In 1980 some local populations of two vectors of the *Simulium damnosum* complex (*S. soubrense* and *S. sanctipauli*) were found to be temephos-resistant and resistance has now spread to other areas. Where it is encountered another organophosphate, chlorphoxim, or the microbial insecticide *Bacillus thuringiensis var. israelensis* (*B.t.i.*) is substituted. There are, however, logistic problems in using this latter insecticide as it does not carry down-stream so far as temephos and considerably greater quantities have to be applied. Despite these and other difficulties, the control scheme has been very successful in greatly reducing onchocerciasis transmission in the OCP area. However, as the worms can live for a very long time in man it seems that control will have to continue for about 20 years.

4 Phlebotomine Sandflies

These insects belong to the subfamily Phlebotominae of the Psychodidae, and comprise some of the smallest insects biting man. They are commonly known as sandflies, because some species breed in sandy areas. However, since very small biting flies called Ceratopogonidae (see Chapter 5) are also occasionally referred to as sandflies (especially in the West Indies and Australia), it is better to distinguish the present insects by calling them phlebotomine sandflies. There are only two medically important genera, *Phlebotomus* which occurs in the Old World tropics but also extends into the Mediterranean region, including Italy, France and Spain, and the genus *Lutzomyia* which is restricted to the New World. A third genus, *Sergentomyia*, occasionally bites man in the Old World tropics but is not a vector.

Adults of all three genera look very similar and it needs a specialist to differentiate between them, but their geographical distribution aids identification. For example if you are bitten by sandflies in South or Central America, they must belong to the genus *Lutzomyia*. The so-called owl midges or moth flies (e.g. *Pericoma* and *Psychoda*), commonly encountered near sewerage works and in damp toilets in northern temperate areas including Britain, are also psychodids and superficially resemble sandflies, but they do not suck blood and are placed in other subfamilies. In addition to a few minor infections, phlebotomine sandflies transmit a group of protozoan diseases called leishmaniasis to man and animals.

4.1 Biology of phlebotomine sandflies

Adults are tiny (1.3–3.5 mm), hairy, yellowish insects with relatively long stilt-like legs and large eyes for their size (Fig. 4-1c). The antennae are filamentous, segmented and pilose (non-feathery) in both sexes. The mouthparts, which are short and rather inconspicuous, project down from the head. The wings are lanceolate and covered in hairs; when the flies are at rest they are held erect over the body. This, and the twice branching vein 2 (visible once the numerous hairs are rubbed from the wing), distinguishes phlebotomine sandflies from the non-biting psychodids (e.g. *Psychoda*).

Females lay minute, ovoid, dark eggs which when microscopically examined are seen to be covered in a sculptured pattern. Oviposition sites include cracks and crevices in soil and masonry, bases of termite mounds, leaf litter, and debris and faeces accumulating in animal shelters. Although eggs may be deposited in what appear to be very dry places, they cannot tolerate desiccation and need a moist microhabitat. Larvae wriggle out

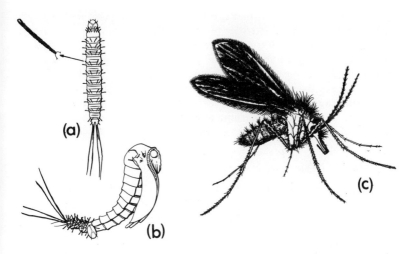

Fig. 4-1 Phlebotomine sandflies: (a) larva with detail of a matchstick hair; (b) pupa with attached larval skin; (c) adult female. (Modified from Smith, 1973. Courtesy British Museum (Nat. Hist.) London.)

from the eggs after 1–2 weeks, but cool weather may delay hatching. Sandfly larvae have small black heads and legless segmented bodies. The presence on the body of thick bristles with feathered stems, in most cases having swollen tips giving rise to the name 'matchstick hairs', and two pairs of conspicuous long caudal bristles, is diagnostic of sandfly larvae (Fig. 4-1a). The larvae are scavengers, feeding on decomposing bodies of small arthropods, animal faeces, fungi and rotting vegetation. There are 4 larval instars. The length of the larval period depends on availability of food, temperature and the species, but is generally completed in 3–8 weeks. In temperate areas sandflies overwinter as diapausing 4th-instar larvae, and may also do so in semi-arid areas during long dry periods. Even in species inhabiting dry regions, the larvae still require a moist microhabitat. Pupae are best recognized by the wrinkled larval skin with its 4 long caudal bristles which, conveniently for entomologists, remains attached to the terminal segments of each pupa (Fig. 4-1b). Pupal duration is about 2–3 weeks.

Adults of both sexes feed on naturally occurring sugary secretions, but in addition females take blood-meals from a variety of vertebrate animals including man, rodents, dogs, foxes, sloths, domestic livestock, reptiles, amphibians and a few species feed on birds. Typically, sandflies bite out of doors in the early evening and during the night, but biting can occur during the daytime, especially when the sky is overcast or if there is forest shade. Some sandflies enter houses to feed and are referred to as domestic or peridomestic species.

Adult sandflies have a characteristic hopping type of flight, consisting of several short flights of about a metre or so before the objective, such as a host, is finally reached. As they are such small and delicate insects, host-seeking and other flight activities cease in the lightest breeze; nevertheless sandflies commonly fly 100 m or more. Biting often occurs in very localized areas, particularly near breeding sites. In Kenya, for example *Phlebotomus martini* bites people mainly near termite mounds which constitute important breeding places. During the day adults shelter in dark and humid sites, including forest vegetation, leaf litter, inbetween buttress roots of large trees, in vent holes of termite mounds, in rodent burrows and caves, and sometimes in houses and animal shelters.

4.2 Medical importance

Although they are such small insects, sandfly bites can be very painful, and have been described as like being stabbed with a red-hot needle. In sensitized people severe irritation can arise from their bites, leading to a condition called Harara in the Middle East.

4.2.1 Leishmaniasis

Phlebotomine sandflies are best known for transmitting several closely related species and strains of protozoans of the genus *Leishmania*. These parasites give rise in man to two main forms of leishmaniasis, namely visceral and cutaneous leishmaniasis.

The rather simple life-cycle of the different *Leishmania* species carried by *Phlebotomus* and *Lutzomyia* vectors is much the same for all species. Intracellular amastigote parasites in a vertebrate host are ingested by a feeding female sandfly and pass to the midgut, where they elongate to become flagellate promastigotes. These forms reproduce by binary fission and migrate to the oesophagous. Five to twelve days after feeding from an infected host, mature infective parasites are present in the vector's mouthparts, and from here they can be injected into a new host when the sandfly takes the next blood-meal. Interestingly, it is believed that if females have previously taken a sugar-meal this somehow enhances the survival and multiplication of the parasites in their guts.

Most forms of leishmaniasis are zoonotic and various wild and domestic animals serve as reservoirs of infection. The degree of involvement of man varies considerably, both geographically and according to the parasite species. Visceral leishmaniasis, often called kala-azar, is caused mainly by *Leishmania donovani*, in the Mediterranean region dogs and foxes are reservoirs and the main vectors are *Phlebotomus perniciosus* and *P. ariasi*. In the Middle East, wild and domestic dogs are important in maintaining the transmission cycle, as they are in China. In South America, domestic and wild canines are important reservoirs, and the vector is *Lutzomyia longipalpis*. In India there is as yet no proven reservoir except man himself, the vector being *Phlebotomus argentipes*.

Cutaneous or dermal leishmaniasis is found in the Indian subregion, the Mediterranean, asiatic Russia, countries of the Near and Middle East and

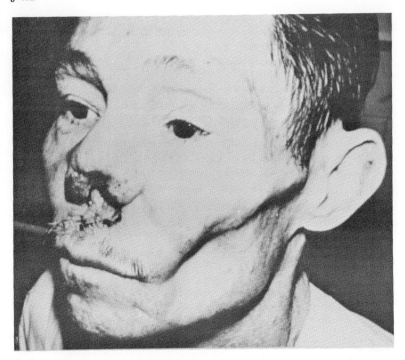

Fig. 4-2 A man from Brazil with his nose partially destroyed by parasites causing mucocutaneous leishmaniasis (Black and white photograph of a colour print in W. Peters and H.M. Gilles, 1977. *A Colour Atlas of Tropical Medicine*, Wolfe Medical Publication, London.)

occasionally in Africa. In these areas the parasites responsible for this form of leishmaniasis are mainly *Leishmania tropica* and *L. major*, and the disease is often called Oriental sore; again rodents are reservoirs. In Central and South America some forms of the disease produce most horrifying disfigurations of the face. The parasites (strains of *L. braziliensis*) attack the mucous membranes, sometimes completely destroying the nose and palate (Fig. 4-2), and this has led to the term mucocutaneous leishmaniasis (espundia). In the Americas, forest rodents, sloths and probably other mammals serve as reservoirs, and an important vector is *Lutzomyia flaviscutella*.

4.2.2 Treatment of leishmaniasis

There are no recognized preventive drugs or vaccines for protection against visceral leishmaniasis. However, a person infected with cutaneous leishmaniasis caused by *L. tropica* usually benefits from life-long immunity, consequently in a few countries, a long-standing custom has been crude inoculation of an arm or leg with a needle contaminated with parasites. This popular practice prevented natural infections and the risks of unsightly marks on the face, especially abhorrent in girls. This practice has, however, been superseded by proper vaccination against *L. tropica*.

Treatment of both visceral and cutaneous leishmaniasis can be prolonged and difficult, for example 30 daily injections with antimonial drugs which often cause undesirable side-effects. Even after such an unpleasant course of treatment there is no guarantee of a cure (see Section 4.3).

4.2.3   Sandfly fever and bartonellosis

A virus disease called sandfly fever, 3-day fever or papatacci fever (so called because the principal vector is *P. patatasi*) occurs in the Mediterranean region, the Near East, parts of the Indian subregion, and possibly elsewhere. As with most vector-borne viral diseases, there is cyclical development in the sandfly and infection is by saliva injected into a host while the sandfly is feeding. There is also transovarial transmission (see Section 1.3.3).

Bartonellosis, sometimes called Carrion's disease or Oroya fever, is cased by the bacteria-like micro-organism *Bartonella bacilliformis*. It is a rare infection encountered only in mountainous regions of Peru, Colombia and Ecuador. Transmission is purely mechanical, being through contaminated mouthparts.

4.3   Vector control

There have been very few campaigns specifically directed against the vectors of leishmaniasis. In India and the Middle East, however, when houses were sprayed with DDT and other insecticides as part of a malaria control campaign, this also resulted in killing domestic phlebotomines and greatly reduced the prevalence of leishmaniasis. Use of very fine bed nets, known as sandfly nets, or better still similar nets impregnated with a residual insecticide, can lessen the chance of being bitten indoors. Catching and destroying dogs, which are important reservoirs, is actively pursued in China, and can assist in reducing transmission.

5 Ceratopogonid Midges

The word midge is commonly applied to many small insects, so to distinguish the ceratopogonids from other so-called midges, including the non-biting chironomids, it is best to refer to them as *biting* midges. They are occasionally called sandflies, a term better restricted to phlebotomines (see chapter 4). Ceratopogonids have a worldwide distribution and are troublesome pests in places as dissimilar as the Scottish highlands and the tropical West Indies. In addition to causing a biting nuisance, they transmit nematode worms to man in a few tropical countries, and in both temperate and tropical areas they are vectors of important livestock diseases such as the bluetongue virus. There are many genera of Ceratopogonidae, but only four contain blood-sucking flies, and of these by far the commonest is *Culicoides*. In the Americas the genus *Leptoconops* also contains troublesome biters which superficially resemble *Culicoides* as well as having a similar biology.

Unless otherwise stated, the following account refers to the genus *Culicoides*, although it is also broadly applicable to *Leptoconops*.

5.1 Biology of *Culicoides*

Adults are very small (1.5–4.5 mm) insects about the same size as phlebotomine sandflies (Chapter 4), and like sandflies they have short inconspicuous mouthparts that hang down from the head (Fig. 5-1c). The antennae are filamentous and segmented, and, as in mosquitoes, are distinctly more hairy in the males. The wings are short and relatively broad, lack scales or conspicuous hairs, but are usually characterized by contrasting blackish and whitish areas which form faint but distinct patterns. (*Leptoconops* differs in having the wings milky white which contrasts sharply with its black body.) The wings are held over the body like the blades of a closed pair of scissors (cf *phlebotomine* sandflies p. 34).

The brownish, and usually banana-shaped, eggs are laid in a variety of wet places including leaf litter, farmyard debris, manure, rotting vegetation, sphagnum bogs, mud of freshwater and saltwater marshes, tree-holes and decaying cut stems of banana plants, while a few *Culicoides* and most *Leptoconops* lay their eggs in coastal sand (hence the name sandflies is often given to ceratopogonids, especially in the West Indies and Australia). Although the immature stages of most *Culicoides* are not aquatic, breeding places are often waterlogged and may even become temporarily flooded. After 2–9 days the eggs hatch to produce minute cylindrical legless larvae, devoid of any obvious characters except for a pair of 4-lobed retractile

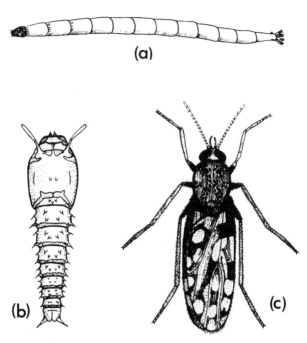

Fig. 5-1 *Culicoides* species: **(a)** larva; **(b)** pupa; **(c)** adult female. (Modified from Service, 1980.)

papillae ('gills') on the last abdominal segment (Fig. 5-1a). There are 4 larval instars. Larvae feed mainly on decaying vegetation. In warm countries the larval period is 2–3 weeks, but in colder temperate areas *Culicoides* overwinter as larvae, and may spend as much as 7 months in this stage. Pupae tend to form in the drier parts of breeding places; they can be recognized by their relatively long respiratory trumpets, which appear to be 2-segmented and by the abdomen being covered in very small tubercles ending in minute setae (Fig. 5-1b). Pupal duration is 3–10 days.

Only female adults take blood-meals and while some species feed exclusively on birds, others feed on various mammals including livestock and man. Biting usually occurs out of doors during the day or night, but adults are especially aggressive in the evenings and during the first half of the night. Like phlebotomine sandflies they have short mouthparts, so biting is restricted to exposed areas of skin, such as around the forehead and hands, or other parts of the body not covered by clothing. Biting is most intense near breeding places, but adults can be dispersed several kilometres by wind, and it has recently been suggested that midges may be blown several hundred kilometres, causing isolated outbreaks of bluetongue virus and African horse sickness.

5.2 Medical and veterinary importance

5.2.1 Biting nuisance

Persistent biting by vast hordes of midges can make outdoor recreational activities and work virtually impossible. In some areas, biting can be so bad as to stop summer harvesting.

5.2.2 Medical vectors

In the West Indies, South America, West and Central Africa and to a much lesser extent in parts of East Africa, *Culicoides* transmits to man the filarial worm *Mansonella perstans* (former generic name, *Dipetalonema* or *Acanthocheilonema*). In the rain forests of West Africa and Zaire a similar parasite, *M. streptocerca*, is also spread to man by *Culicoides*, and *M. ozzardi*, is transmitted by *Culicoides* in the West Indies and parts of Central and South America. The method of transmission is basically the same for all species and is similar to that described for filarial infections carried by mosquitoes (p. 18). Summarized briefly, microfilariae, in these instances non-periodic forms, are taken up from the blood (*M. perstans*, *M. ozzardi*) or skin (*M. streptocerca*) when the female flies are feeding. In the fly, they undergo cyclical development in the thoracic flight muscles resulting in infective larvae appearing in the insect's proboscis after 6–10 days. On feeding again, a few infective worms are deposited on a person's skin. In Africa, especially West Africa, the most important vectors of worms are *Culicoides austeni* and *C. grahamii*, both of which breed in the rotting stumps of banana plants. *C. furens* is a common vector of *M. ozzardi* in the Caribbean (see also p. 33). None of these filarial parasites appears to cause much, if any, harm to man. In Brazil *C. paraensis* is a vector of Oropouche virus, the only known virus transmitted to man by *Culicoides*.

In summary *Culicoides* are not generally regarded as important medically, except that their biting can sometimes be intolerable.

5.2.3 Veterinary vectors

Bluetongue fever is an important viral disease of sheep spread by *Culicoides*. It can cause serious economic losses and is found in many parts of the world, but not in Britain. Other *Culicoides* transmitted viral diseases include bovine ephemeral fever of cattle in Africa and Australia, and African horse sickness. Other less important veterinary parasites transmitted by midges include the filarial worm *Onchocerca cervicalis*, *O. gibsoni* of horses, and a few protozoan parasites of wild animals and poultry, such as *Haemoproteus nettionis* of ducks and geese.

5.3 Control

There are no very effective control measures to reduce attacks by midges, partly because larval habitats can be very difficult to find; they may be very localized, or may extend over large areas. An additional difficulty is that very large volumes of insecticidal solution must be applied to ensure that it is washed down through the soil, leaf litter, mud etc. to reach the larvae buried underneath the surface. The most suitable insecticides are the persistent organochlorines such as DDT and dieldrin, but these are environmentally unacceptable. Instead, biodegradable organophosphates and carbamates are usually recommended, though they are less effective. Fogging areas with insecticides can give some immediate but temporary relief against biting adults. Repellents smeared over the face and hands and other exposed parts of the body can also afford some degree of protection.

6 Tabanids

The family Tabanidae includes the largest flies biting man or animals. There are many genera, but the medically important ones are *Tabanus* and *Haematopota*, and more especially *Chrysops*, which in Africa transmits filarial worms causing a disease called loiasis. *Chrysops* and *Tabanus* have a worldwide distribution, but *Haematopota* is absent from Australia and South America, and is uncommon in North America. *Chrysops* are sometimes known as deer flies, *Haematopota* are called clegs, while the Tabanidae as a whole, but commonly just the genus *Tabanus*, are known as horseflies.

6.1 Biology of tabanids

Tabanids are large (5–25 mm long), robust, strong flying insects, the largest being certain species of *Tabanus* which have a wing span of 6.5 cm. *Chrysops* and *Tabanus* have brown, black, yellow, reddish, or green bodies, often with conspicuous abdominal stripes. In contrast, *Haematopota* is covered in grey and black markings. Tabanids have large semicircular heads bearing a pair of conspicuous large eyes which usually have iridescent zigzags or bands of bright colours; these colours tend to fade after death. The males, which do not bite, have holoptic eyes (i.e. the eyes join, or nearly join, along the top of the head; simuliid males also have holoptic eyes see p. 29). In females the eyes are dichoptic (that is, they are separate), this is most easily seen in *Chrysops*. The mouthparts hang down from the head and are relatively short, but are stout and blunt-tipped. The antennae are three-segmented; length and shape are variable. The wings are broad, without scales or hairs, but have very distinct veins. The following notes will help distinguish between adults of the three most important genera.

Chrysops   These are medium-sized flies (6–10 mm long). The wings usually have one or two brownish transverse bands, and are held like an open pair of scissors over the body. The antennae are markedly longer than in the other genera and each is composed of 3 similar segments (Fig. 6-1b).

Haematopota   These are medium-sized flies (6–10 mm long), having a distinctly dusty appearance due to mottling of grey and black markings on both wings and body. Unlike other genera the wings are held roof-like over the body. The antennae are similar to those of *Tabanus*, but the 3rd segment is not upturned and lacks a dorsal projection (Fig. 6-1d).

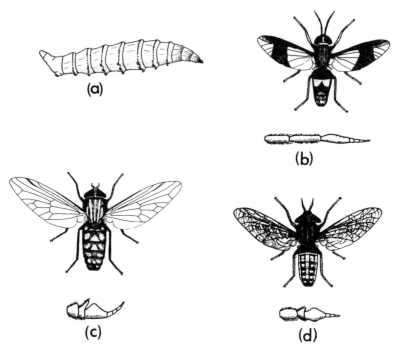

Fig. 6-1 Tabanids: (**a**) larva; (**b**) adult females and antennae of *Chrysops*; (**c**) *Tabanus*; (**d**) *Haematopota*. (Modified from Service, 1980.)

Tabanus   These are medium to large flies (9–25 mm long), usually with clear wings held 'open scissor-fashion' over the body. The antennae are short, the 2nd and 3rd segments have small dorsal projections and the 3rd segment usually curves upwards (Fig. 6-1c).

Tabanids lay from several to many hundred cigar-shaped eggs. These are glued onto vegetation, stones or rocks overhanging larval habitats, often in a lozenge- or rhomboid-shaped pattern. Larvae hatch from the eggs after 1–2 weeks and drop down onto the underlying mud, damp soil or water. The larvae are creamy white, cylindrical and pointed at both ends. Posteriorly each has a short conical siphon through which it breathes. The larvae are readily identified by conspicuous tyre-like rings which encircle the body and by having 6 round protuberances called pseudopods placed ventrolaterally on most segments (Fig. 6-1a). Fully grown tabanid larvae can measure 1–6 cm. They live in damp soil, in mud at edges of fresh or salt-water marshes, ponds and ditches, in rotting vegetation and debris, and in shallow water at the edge of pools or streams. A few species inhabit drier soils, especially at the base of trees, a habitat reminiscent of that of tsetse fly puparia (p. 48).

Larvae of most species of *Tabanus* and *Haematopota* feed on soil-inhabiting arthropods; a few are cannibalistic. *Chrysops* larvae, and those of a few *Tabanus* and *Haematopota* species, feed on dead and decaying vegetable and animal remains. Larval duration is long. Even in tropical countries it is 4–5 months and may sometimes be a year or more, while in temperate areas larval development may extend to 2 or more years. Pupation occurs in drier areas of the larval habitat, and the brown pupae superficially resemble the chrysalids of butterflies. Adults emerge from the pupae after 1–3 weeks.

Most tabanids live in woods and forests, but some, especially *Chrysops*, are common in marshy areas, while others frequent more open savannas and grasslands. Only females are blood-sucking. Most species feed during the daytime – sight is important in host location, females being particularly attracted to dark moving objects. Tabanids will follow slowly driven vehicles and enter through the windows and will also alight on the tyres when the vehicle has stopped and attempt to feed – being dark and warm the tyres are mistaken for hosts! People are usually bitten on the back of the body and legs, and caucasians are frequently bitten through dark clothing in preference to exposed areas of pale skin. Because of their blunt mouth-parts tabanids inflict painful bites, and this often causes them to be disturbed before they have taken a full blood-meal.

Typically tabanids feed out of doors, but some species, including the African filarial vector *Chrysops silacea*, may enter well-lit houses to bite. In addition to man, large wild and domestic animals such as deer, cattle and horses are frequently pestered by tabanids.

In temperate countries, adult tabanids are markedly seasonal. In Britain, for instance, biting is usually only intense during July and August. In tropical countries breeding is normally continuous, but nevertheless biting populations are usually largest at the beginning of the rainy season.

6.2 Medical and veterinary importance

Tabanids can be annoying pests, but luckily in many places, the biting season is short. In Japan tabanid *larvae* are said to bite the feet of people working in the ricefields and cause oedema.

Because of their coarse mouthparts and frequency of interrupted feeding (see Section 1.3.1), tabanids are efficient mechanical vectors of some diseases. For example, they can transmit tularaemia which is caused by *Francisella tularensis*, a bacterial disease that infects man, rabbits and rodents, and is spread by a variety of methods, including tick bites and insufficiently cooked meat. Tabanids can also be mechanical vectors of anthrax and the protozoan parasite *Trypanosoma evansi*, that affects camels, horses and dogs, sometimes with fatal results. Tabanids also cyclically transmit *T. theileri* to cattle and antelopes. In Africa they may play a *very minor* role in transmitting human and animal trypanosomiasis, the principal vectors being tsetse flies (see Chapter 7). In South America, where there are no tsetse flies, *Trypanosoma vivax*, an important parasite of cattle, is probably spread mechanically by tabanids.

It is, however, the role of certain species of *Chrysops* as vectors of the filarial parasite *Loa loa* that makes the Tabanidae of some medical importance. Occuring mainly in West Africa, but also to a limited extent in Central Africa, loiasis is essentially a disease encountered in humid forests. It is transmitted by day-biting *Chrysops silacea* and *C. dimidiata*. Diurnally periodic microfilariae of *L. loa* are picked up from the blood when females are biting, and 10–12 days later, having undergone cyclical development in the fly's thoracic muscles, infective larvae are present in the fly's proboscis. A new host becomes infected when a few larvae are deposited on the skin during feeding.

Loiasis is famous for two clinical symptoms, namely, itchy lumps on the arms and body called Calabar swellings (named after the town in eastern Nigeria), and the alarming sight of a worm crossing the eye under the conjunctiva! Its thrashing journey takes about half an hour, but apart from shock and intense irritation no real harm is done by this migration.

6.3   Treatment and control of loiasis

Both adult worms (which can live in man for 18 or more years) and microfilariae are killed by oral administration over 3 weeks of a drug called DEC (diethylcarbamazine). Side-reactions such as fever and headache commonly occur, but are not usually serious.

Control of *Chrysops* vectors is not economically practical, and only limited protection from their bites can be achieved by applying repellents like diethyltoluamide and dimethylphthalate.

7 Tsetse Flies

Tsetse flies occupy some 10 million km² of Africa (almost half of the continent), mostly between latitudes 15° north and 20° south. They are of great veterinary importance as vectors of trypanosome parasites causing nagana, or animal trypanosomiasis, in cattle and other domestic animals, and are locally important as vectors of sleeping sickness.

There are only 22 species of tsetse flies, all of which belong to *Glossina*, a genus restricted to Africa. They have played an historic role, mainly as vectors of nagana, in hindering the development and exploitation of tropical Africa. In the past, nagana prevented the use of draught animals in ploughing and of horses as pack animals, and today the disease still limits agricultural development. There have also been some devastating sleeping sickness epidemics in Africa, for example, between 1900 and 1906 it caused the death of an estimated 0.25 million Ugandans, and even today outbreaks can result in many thousands dying.

7.1 Biology of tsetse flies

Adults are medium to large (6–15 mm), brownish insects being a little bigger than houseflies. They can be distinguished from other biting flies by possession of a forwardly projecting proboscis having a basal bulb-like swelling, and by wing veins 4 and 5 enclosing a 'cell' that with a little imagination resembles an upside down hatchet or chopper (Fig. 7-1c): not surprisingly it is called the 'hatchet cell'. Tsetse flies also differ from most other similar sized flies in folding their wings over the body like the closed blades of a pair of scissors; in houseflies and most other flies the wings remain apart like the blades of an open pair of scissors. Epidemiologically it is not necessary to sex tsetse flies because both males and females suck blood, nevertheless males can be recognized by a rather prominent raised circular knob-like structure on the underside of the tip of the abdomen comprising the external genitalia.

In contrast to most flies, tsetse flies do not lay eggs but deposit a single larva at the end of each reproductive cycle, that is, they are viviparous. When an egg is mature it passes down the oviduct, is fertilized by one of the spermatozoa stored in the paired spermothecae, and after 3–5 days, hatches. The resultant larva lives in the uterus and is nourished by secretions of the so-called 'milk' or accessory glands, and after 4–5 days the larva (8–9 mm) is ready to be discharged. During larval development the female takes a blood-meal about every 2–3 days. If she is unable to find suitable hosts, the ill-nourished larva is aborted. A tsetse fly harbouring a more or less fully grown larva is easily recognized by her greatly enlarged abdomen; she is referred to as being 'pregnant'.

The larva is born posterior end first – so it is a 'breech case' – and is deposited amongst loose, friable soil or sand underneath trees, bushes, fallen logs, between buttress roots of trees, in river beds or in animal burrows. It is segmented, creamy white, rather bullet-shaped and has two black conspicuous polyneustic lobes (Fig. 7-1a), which are respiratory. It immediately buries into the loose earth. Within about 20 minutes the integument hardens and, as in houseflies, a barrel-shaped dark brown puparium is formed. Tsetse puparia are distinguished by their dark polyneustic lobes (Fig. 7-1c). Tsetse flies remain as puparia for 4–5 weeks, after which the adults emerge.

A female tsetse fly produces a larva about every 9–12 days and during her lifetime probably deposits a total of 5–8 larvae. The reproductive rate of tsetse flies is therefore very low, but this is to some extent compensated for by the high survival rate of the immature stages; nevertheless tsetse populations are rarely very large.

Most species have definite host preferences, for example *Glossina swynnertoni* of East Africa, feeds preferentially on wild pigs, while *G. morsitans* in East Africa feeds mainly on wild and domestic bovids as well as wild suids, whereas in West Africa, warthogs are its favourite hosts. The West African *G. palpalis* feeds predominantly on reptiles. These three species will also bite man and are in fact, efficient vectors of human trypanosomiasis. Feeding is restricted to the daytime and as with tabanids, vision is important in host seeking, dark moving objects being especially attractive. Again like tabanids, tsetse flies prefer to bite through dark coloured clothing rather than exposed skin of pale-skinned people. Tsetse flies rest in shaded sites to avoid high temperatures (above 36°C) and dry environments. Favoured daytime resting sites include the underside of thick twigs and branches, and trunks of trees up to a height of about 4 m. At night many species tend to rest on the upper surface of leaves and thin twigs. Knowledge of resting sites is relevant to tsetse control operations (p. 53).

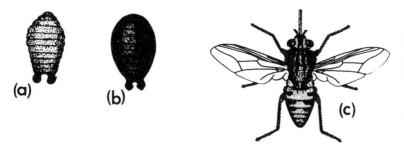

Fig. 7-1   Tsetse flies: (a) larva; (b) puparium; (c) adult fly. (Modified from Service, 1980.)

Breeding is continuous throughout the year. Maximum populations are encountered at the end of the rainy season. During dry periods, when suitable resting places for flies and larviposition sites become restricted, populations are reduced.

7.1.1   Tsetse groups

Based on morphological characters and on their ecology and distribution, tsetse flies can be divided into the following three main groups.

Fusca group (forest flies)   This group inhabits equatorial rain forests and contains the largest tsetse flies, up to 15.5 mm in length. *Glossina fusca* is a typical West African example, while *G. brevipalpis* is a common East African forest fly. The flies in this group do not transmit sleeping sickness because they very rarely bite man, but they are important vectors of nagana to cattle.

Morsitans group (savanna flies)   These flies live in the relatively dry savanna areas, including thicket vegetation and grassland; they may extend to semi-desert regions. *G. morsitans* is a common species in West, Central and East Africa and a most important sleeping sickness vector. Other vectors include *G. pallidipes* and *G. swynnertoni*, both of which are restricted to East African savannas.

Palpalis group (riverine flies)   These flies are found in wetter vegetation, such as that growing along river banks and bordering lakes, and are sometimes encountered in forests and mangrove swamps. *G. palpalis* is the commonest species in West Africa, its counterpart in East and Central Africa being *G. fuscipes*. Another common species, *G. tachinoides*, is found mainly in West Africa, but also occurs in Central Africa and in Ethiopia. All three species transmit sleeping sickness.

7.2   Medical importance

Trypanosoma brucei gambiense causes sleeping sickness, or human trypanosomiasis, in West Africa, and the closely related and morphologically indistinguishable *T. brucei rhodesiense* is responsible for the East African form of sleeping sickness. Although the parasites are morphologically identical (they are differentiated by biochemical methods, including electrophoresis), the epidemiology and clinical symptoms of these two forms of sleeping sickness are distinct.

The cycle of development in the tsetse fly of both trypanosome species (and also *T. brucei brucei* which causes animal trypanosomiasis) is the same, and is as follows. Trypanosomes (amastigotes), ingested by male or female flies while feeding on man or animal reservoirs, pass to the stomach. Here they multiply and then start their migration by a rather complicated route to reach the tsetse fly's long and thread-like salivary glands. There is still controversy as to the exact migratory path followed by the parasites, but essentially they pass from the gut to the space between the peritrophic membrane and stomach. From here they pass into the proventriculus and travel to the tip of the proboscis where they reverse their direction of travel and return up the hypopharynx to reach the salivary glands. This journey takes 18–34 days. Laboratory evidence suggests that parasites might be able to pass across the stomach wall into the haemocoele and then directly enter the salivary glands. Whether this much simpler route occurs in field populations, and if so, how important it is, has not been established. Parasites in the salivary glands, called trypomastigotes, are injected into a new host when a tsetse fly feeds, and thus a new infection is established.

7.2.1   Gambian sleeping sickness

This is caused by *T. brucei gambiense* and is transmitted chiefly by *G. palpalis* and *G. tachinoides* in West Africa, and in Central Africa and parts of East Africa by *G. fuscipes*. These riverine flies are especially common at watering places, fords across rivers and along lake shores, and consequently fishermen and women washing clothes in streams are particularly liable to infection. Animal reservoirs are probably less important than for *T.b. rhodesiense*, but there is evidence that domestic pigs and some wild mammals may harbour *T.b. gambiense*.

Trypanosomes are found in the blood and in the lymph glands. An early symptom of infection is enlarged glands at the base of the neck. (In 1803 T.M. Winterbottom, a physician in West Africa, drew attention to the fact that slave traders rejected potential slaves showing such swollen glands, because they knew they were unlikely to survive the long journey from West Africa to the New World.) Towards the beginning of an infection there may occasionally be spontaneous recovery, but more usually, after some months or a year or more of low-grade symptoms, the parasites invade the central nervous system. This causes lethargy and psychiatric complications, and eventually the person stops eating and sleeps virtually all the time (Fig. 7-2), and some months later dies.

7.2.2   Rhodesian sleeping sickness

This is a much more virulent disease than the Gambian form. The causative agent, *T. brucei rhodesiense*, is transmitted mainly by *G. morsitans*; other vectors include *G. swynnertoni* and *G. pallidipes*. All three tsetse species also feed on game animals, some of which are reservoir hosts of Rhodesian sleeping sickness, which is a zoonotic disease with man as a secondary host. Hunters, charcoal burners, honey-gatherers and pastoralists who spend much of their time in savanna areas are at special risk of infection, as are tourists visiting game reserves.

Infected people may die before the central nervous system is affected. However, when trypanosomes invade the cerebrospinal fluid the clinical symptoms are much as for Gambian sleeping sickness, namely lethargy and sleepiness, but death comes more quickly, usually after only a few weeks.

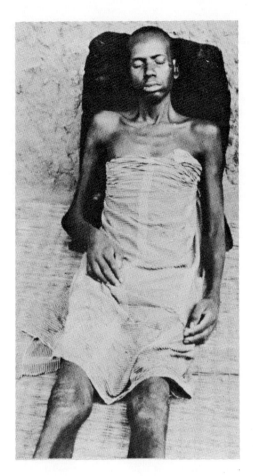

Fig. 7-2 A person in West Africa suffering from advanced stages of Gambian type sleeping sickness (D. Scott.)

7.2.3   Treatment of sleeping sickness

With early diagnosis, treatment consists of injections with pentamidine or suramin given over a number of days. The latter drug, however, can produce unpleasant side-reactions. When the central nervous system is affected a series of injections with arsenical compounds such as melarsoprol is necessary, but this is a dangerous drug and up to 5% of those treated die from its toxic effects.

A single intramuscular injection of pentamidine can provide protection against *T. b. gambiense* for up to 6 months, but there is no recommended prophylaxis against the Rhodesian form. There are instances of drug resistance, but this is a more serious problem in the chemotherapy of animal trypanosomiasis.

7.3 Nagana or animal trypanosomiasis

Four species of trypanosomes cause nagana in cattle; *T. brucei brucei* (morphologically identical to the parasites responsible for sleeping sickness), *T. congolense*, *T. vivax* and *T. simiae*. The cyclical development in the tsetse fly of the latter three species differs from the *brucei* group trypanosomes, in that the infective forms are found not in the salivary glands but in the proboscis. All four parasites occur in game animals such as antelopes, where they do little, if any harm, but infected cattle give greatly reduced milk yields, become sick and emaciated and often die. Local herdsmen can often recognize fly-infested areas, the so-called 'fly-belts', and try to avoid them. Animal trypanosomiasis remains one of the more serious veterinary diseases in Africa, and still prevents efficient cattle ranching in a continent that urgently needs more protein. Economically, trypanosomiasis of cattle is more important than human trypanosomiasis. Three strategies are adopted to reduce nagana.

(*a*) Prophylactic drugs can give cattle some degree of protection, but repeated treatments are necessary, and only the richer farmers can afford this. Drug resistant strains of trypanosomes are becoming increasingly common and pose a serious problem.

(*b*) Some cattle breeds, such as the N'dama and Muturu of West Africa, are less susceptible to trypanosomiasis than other breeds. Even so, such trypanotolerant breeds still deteriorate if exposed to dense populations of tsetse flies.

(*c*) Control measures may be aimed at reducing the numbers of tsetse flies, but this approach is used much less in combating nagana than in the attempted control of sleeping sickness; insecticides are relied upon heavily in this control (see Section 7.4).

7.4 Tsetse fly control

Because game animals are reservoirs of Rhodesian sleeping sickness, they were formerly slaughtered indiscriminately in eastern Africa, but such widespread destruction of wildlife is no longer acceptable.

Another method is the selective removal of vegetation which provides resting sites, shade and moisture for adult tsetse flies. This approach relies on good knowledge of the biology of the flies. Bush clearance, as it is often called, has in the past been very successful, but is now little practiced as it has been superseded by the use of insecticides. It has also become increasingly costly in terms of labour, and is often regarded as ecologically undesirable.

The use of insecticides provides the main strategy for tsetse control, and fortunately tsetse flies have not yet evolved insecticide resistance. The organochlorine insecticides DDT and dieldrin are selectively sprayed onto resting sites, such as tree trunks up to a height of about 1.5 m in the dry season or 3.5 m in the wet season. Aerial spraying can give effective control over large areas. This involves using either non-residual formulations of endosulfan or synthetic pyrethroids like deltamethrin applied from fixed-wing aircraft, or residual formulations of insecticides such as dieldrin and endosulfan from helicopters. Although residual applications from the air kill more non-target organisms than selective ground spraying, non-residual aerial spraying kills very many less. Repeated treatments of non-residual insecticides are essential, because a large proportion of the tsetse population at the time of spraying is composed of puparia, which lie concealed beneath the soil and thus remain unaffected.

Undoubtedly insecticidal spraying causes environmental damage but after an area has been cleared of flies and spraying has terminated, it will usually become recolonized by most wild life.

8 Fleas

Fleas belong to the order Siphonaptera. They have a worldwide distribution and comprise some 3000 species, 94% of which are ectoparasites on mammals, the remainder on birds. The human flea, *Pulex irritans*, was formerly a common household pest and plague vector, but is now uncommon. This was the flea that was trained to pull miniscule silver carriages, ride bicycles and perform other fascinating feats in flea circuses, which were still being performed in Britain in 1976. In temperate regions the most troublesome fleas are generally cat and dog fleas (*Ctenocephalides felis* and *C. canis*), but it is as vectors of plague – the infamous Black Death of the 14th century – that fleas have gained notoriety.

8.1 Biology of fleas

Adults are small (1–4 mm), wingless, brownish insects, flattened laterally and covered in backward-pointing bristles (Fig. 8-1c). The head is roughly triangular and usually has a pair of conspicuous black eyes, a pair of small antennae lying in grooves, and ventrally there may be a row of coarse teeth forming the genal comb or ctenidium. The mouthparts are short and directed downwards. The first thoracic segment may bear a pronotal comb (similar to the genal comb). The flea's legs are long, especially the hind pair which are used for jumping; human fleas can jump 20 cm vertically and 30 cm or more horizontally, a remarkable feat for such small creatures! Male fleas can be recognized by the upturned tips of their abdomens, but as both sexes take blood-meals, sexing fleas is not very important.

Eggs are laid in debris that accumulates in the host's nest or burrow, or in the case of cat and dog fleas in cracks and crevices in floors or on carpets. The white and rather sticky eggs hatch after about 2–14 days. The larva (Fig. 8-1a) has a black head and a brown segmented body covered in fine setae. Two papillae on the last abdominal segment, called anal struts, immediately identify flea larvae. They shelter in cracks and crevices and feed on organic debris, including animal faeces and spots of dried blood discharged by adult fleas. The larval period usually lasts 2–3 weeks, but if temperatures are low and food is scarce, this may be extended to 200 days or more. Finally, the larva spins a silken cocoon which soon becomes camouflaged with debris, after a few days the larva inside the cocoon pupates (Fig. 8-1b). Adults are formed after 1–2 weeks, but they require a stimulus, such as vibrations caused by animal movements, before they escape from their cocoons. If there is no suitable stimulus adults can remain alive in their cocoons for a year. This explains why people entering houses

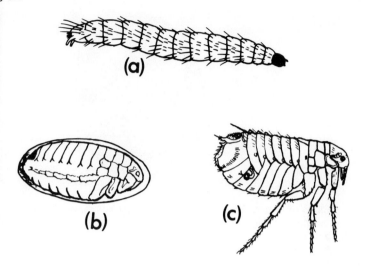

Fig. 8-1   Life-cycle of a typical flea: **(a)** larva; **(b)** cocoon containing pupa; **(c)** adult female flea. (Modified from Service, 1980.)

that have been empty for months may be suddenly bitten by numerous hungry fleas.

Fleas are very active and generally avoid light. For example, when fleas are exposed during searches on cats or dogs they rapidly run down to the base of the fur. They can be caught by dabbing them with sellotape or a matchstick smeared with glue or vaseline. Fleas are sometimes found hiding in beds or under clothing.

In a typical infestation a cat may harbour only 25 fleas, but there may be several hundred in its bedding and favourite sleeping quarters around the house. In addition there are probably as many as 500 cocoons and 3000 larvae on the floor. Vacuum cleaning carpets undoubtedly destroys many fleas, and helps maintain low populations.

Fleas feed several times during the day or night. Although they exhibit host preferences, most will feed on alternative hosts. For example, both cat and dog fleas (*Ctenocephalides felis* and *C. canis*) readily attack man, especially when there are heavy infestations, or pets leave home or die. The human flea, *Pulex irritans*, also feeds on pigs. Fleas vacate dead animals and this has great epidemiological significance in plague transmission (p. 57).

8.2   Life-cycle of the chigoe flea

The chigoe, jigger or sand flea, *Tunga penetrans*, originated in South America but has now spread to several tropical regions, including Africa. It is not indigenous in Asia, although people returning from overseas

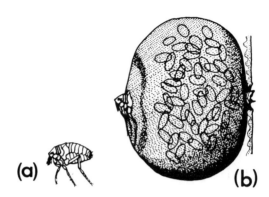

Fig. 8-2 Adults of chigoe flea (*Tunga penetrans*): (a) non-gravid female flea; (b) female imbedded in skin and having enormously swollen abdomen containing eggs. (Modified from Service, 1980.)

may be infected.

Adults (Fig. 8-2a) are only about 1 mm long and the three thoracic segments are greatly compressed. As with all fleas both sexes take blood-meals, the favoured hosts being man and pigs, but unlike other fleas the fertilized female buries into the skin, mainly between the toes, and remains there throughout her life. Only the extreme tip of her abdomen is exposed (8-2b). Beggars, infants and leprosy patients who habitually sit on the ground often have the buttocks infested with chigoe fleas. The area around the embedded flea becomes red and itchy and secondary infections may occur. After a little more than a week, the flea's abdomen becomes greatly swollen (6 mm) and she starts discharging large numbers of eggs. These fall onto the floors of houses or on the ground outside, where after 3–4 days they hatch, and as in other fleas the larvae eventually spin their cocoons and pupate. After 1–2 weeks the flea stops laying eggs and dies *in situ*. Not surprisingly this frequently causes inflammation, ulceration and secondary infections, and in extreme cases tetanus may arise, and toes may be lost due to gangrene.

As the chigoe flea is a poor jumper, wearing shoes greatly reduces the chance of becoming infected. Sterile needles should be used to remove embedded fleas; local people are often adept at removing fleas, but not usually under aseptic conditions!

8.3 Other fleas

A very small flea (1 mm) called *Echidnophaga gallinacea* can become a serious pest of poultry in subtropical and tropical countries. Adults of both sexes bury their mouthparts more or less permanently into the neck and head of poultry and sometimes wild birds. Heavy infestations can lead to anaemia and emaciation, reduced egg laying and death of young birds. These fleas, commonly referred to as sticktight fleas, very occasionally become attached to man, but apart from some discomfort they do no harm.

Most mammals and many birds have their own species of fleas, but they usually appear to cause them little harm apart from annoyance and irritation.

8.4   Medical importance

8.4.1   Nuisance

Fleas can constitute a biting nuisance almost anywhere. In many countries the major problem arises from fleas of household pets attacking their owners. Fleas mostly bite the ankles and lower legs (wearing sticky gaiters when visiting flea-infested premises not only prevents one getting bitten, but catches a good sample of fleas!) Fleas will, however, bite any part of the body when you are in bed.

8.4.2   Plague

The causative agent of bubonic plague is a bacterium called *Yersinia (Pasteurella) pestis* which is spread by fleas. Within recent history there have been three plague pandemics, the first began in the 6th century in Arabia and spread to Turkey, Europe and North Africa. The second pandemic originated in Asia and spread eastwards to China, southwards to India and westwards into Europe where it caused the infamous Black Death (1349–51). The third pandemic started in 1892 in China and rapidly spread to Hong Kong and then to India, Africa, Australia, California and to South America. The plague of London of 1665 mentioned by Samuel Pepys in his diary was also due to *Y. pestis*.

Bubonic plague is primarily a disease of wild animals, particularly rodents, and is transmitted by many species of fleas. This constitutes the sylvatic or rural cycle of plague. Occasionally hunters become infected with plague through being bitten by rodent fleas, but more usually, domestic rats become infected from this reservoir of sylvatic plague. Rat fleas of the genus *Xenopsylla* then spread the disease amongst rat populations. Rats, especially *Rattus rattus*, live in close association with man, and when they die, often because of plague, their fleas jump onto man and the human population becomes infected. This is known as the urban cycle of plague transmission.

Infection with plague is through the bite of the flea. After a flea has ingested plague-contaminated blood the bacilli multiply enormously in its stomach, and then invade the proventriculus which becomes partially or completely blocked with bacilli. When such fleas try to feed again, the host's blood is sucked up as far as the proventriculus, but as it cannot enter the stomach it is regurgitated into the host, along with plague bacilli. These 'blocked' fleas are particularly dangerous, because as they cannot ingest a blood-meal they repeatedly bite, so a single flea often infects several people.

A less important method of transmission is by the flea's faeces being scratched into cuts and abrasions. Plague bacilli can remain viable in the flea's faeces for up to 3 years.

Plague victims develop a high temperature and skin rash, vomit and frequently experience comas and convulsions. The most characteristic symptom, however, is the development of swollen and hardened lymph glands, especially in the groin, which are termed buboes – hence the name bubonic plague. The death rate from untreated plague patients ranges from 60–95%, but plague is readily cured with sulphonamides or antibiotic drugs and vaccination against plague is available.

Another less common form of plague, called pneumonic plague, is spread not by fleas but by respiratory droplets.

8.4.3   Other flea-transmitted infections

Rickettsiae are bacteria-like organisms and one species, *Rickettsia mooseri* which causes flea-borne typhus, is transmitted from rodents to man by flea faeces infecting cuts and abrasions. Under ideal conditions the rickettsiae can remain viable in the faeces for 9 years. Flea-borne typhus is a relatively mild disease, but patients develop a high temperature and a rash; death is unusual except in people over 50 years of age.

Very occasionally tapeworms, such as *Dipylidium caninum* of dogs and cats, are transmitted to man by fleas. Briefly, the cycle is as follows. Tapeworm eggs in the dog's faeces are eaten by flea larvae, they hatch and the parasites pass onto the adult fleas. If these are swallowed by children kissing and fondling pets, infection can occur. Infections usually produce no symptoms.

Myxomatosis, a virulent viral infection of rabbits, often causing their death, is spread mechanically by rabbit fleas (*Spilopsyllus cuniculi*).

8.5   Flea control

Propriety insecticides can be applied to domestic pets to kill fleas. Plastic collars impregnated with the fumigant insecticide dichlorvos (DDVP) placed round cats' necks are, however, not very effective. It is better to apply insecticide like DDT, HCH, malathion, diazinon, or carbaryl to the sleeping quarters as this is where the flea numbers are greatest. Treatment is repeated after 2 weeks, and may have to be continued for many months to eradicate fleas. Insecticidal dusts can be blown down animal burrows or placed in their runs to kill rodent fleas; premises infested with rats can be fogged with insecticidal aerosols. In urban plague situations, baits poisoned with anticoagulants and slow-acting rodenticides such as warfarin and fumarin are often used to kill commensal rats. Alternatively, dangerous poisons such as strychnine and sodium fluoroacetate, the so-called 'one-dose' poisons, can be used to achieve rapid kills. It is advisable to kill the fleas before killing the rodents, or fleas abandoning dead rats may turn to man, which will enhance plague transmission.

9 Lice

There are two main types of lice: chewing lice belonging to the order Mallophaga which do not infest man, but are common on many mammals and birds; and blood-sucking lice of the order Anoplura. The latter contain several genera (e.g. *Haematopinus*) having species which suck blood from domestic and wild mammals, and three species which are ectoparasites on man. These are the head louse *Pediculus humanus capitis*, the morphologically almost identical body louse *Pediculus humanus humanus*, and the different looking pubic louse *Pthirus pubis*. In the laboratory, head and body lice can be induced to interbreed, but there is very little evidence that natural hybridization occurs. Lice found on the head can be regarded as head lice and those on clothing as body lice.

Lice are the commonest ectoparasites of man, and until fairly recent times most people probably had lice. Even today, head lice are quite common in children in Europe and North America as well as in the developing world; pubic lice are also common. The louse of medical importance is the body louse, which is a vector of epidemic typhus.

9.1 Biology of lice

9.1.1 *Body lice* (Pediculus humanus humanus)

The biology of body and head lice is similar, and although this account refers to the body louse, much of it is also applicable to head lice, except for a few differences outlined in the next section.

Adults are small (3–4.5 mm), greyish, wingless insects that are flattened dorsoventrally (Fig. 9-1c). Their biting mouthparts are unusual in that they do not form a projecting proboscis. Instead, the mouth is tube-like and armed apically with teeth which grip the host's skin. Needle-like stylets are thrust forward to pierce the skin, and blood is sucked into the tubular mouth and passed to the stomach. The legs are stout and end in two claws (comprising a short tibial spine and a longer tarsal claw) which enable lice to hold onto the host. The tip of the female abdomen is bifurcated, but as both sexes suck blood, differentiating between the sexes is not important. Adults cling mostly to the hairs of clothing and only attach themselves to body hairs when feeding, which occurs during both day and night.

The female louse glues her eggs, commonly called nits, onto hairs of clothing (Fig. 9-1a), especially those along the seams of underclothing and woollen materials; more rarely eggs are attached to body hairs. The oval white eggs have a distinct operculum perforated with minute holes through which the embryo breathes. Just before hatching, air entering through the

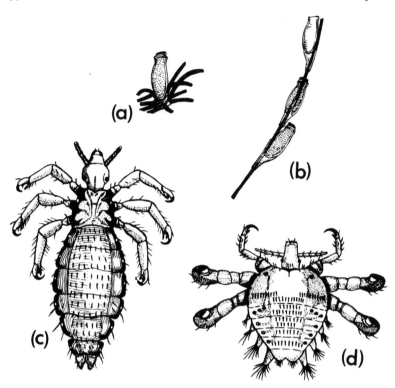

Fig. 9-1 Lice: (**a**) egg of body louse on cloth fibres; (**b**) eggs of head louse on hair from head; (**c**) body louse; (**d**) pubic louse. (From Service, 1980.)

operculum is swallowed by the nymph inside the egg and is passed out through its anus. This builds up a back-pressure, forcing the nymph against the operculum which is consequently pushed off. Hatching occurs after about a week, or if the clothing is discarded, after 2–3 weeks. The life-cycle is hemimetabolous and the 3 nymphal stages are miniature editions of the adult; they suck blood and after 1–2 weeks become adults. If, however, the clothing is removed at night and subjected to low temperatures, the nymphal stage is extended. Lice live only a few days away from their hosts; unfed adults die after 2–5 days, but recently engorged ones might survive for up to 10 days. Lice are sensitive to extreme temperatures, vacating someone with a feverish temperature (40°C or more) and rapidly crawling away from a dead person. It is said that body lice marched like a retreating army from the slaughtered body of Thomas Beckett as it lay in Westminister Abbey.

Body lice are common on people who rarely change their clothing (washing clothes in hot water and ironing kills lice); vagrants are commonly infested with them. Lice are spread by close contact, especially when people are living and sleeping together in crowded conditions, such as troops living in trenches and people in refugee camps and prisons. They are commonly spread during disasters such as floods, earthquakes and famines which force people to live communally. For obvious reasons body lice are more common in cool climates.

In exceptional cases a person may have several hundred lice, and there is a record of a shirt having an estimated 10 000 lice and 10 000 eggs! Usually, however, the number of lice on a person is much less than one hundred.

9.1.2 *Head lice* (Pediculus humanus capitis)

The biology of head lice is much as for body lice, except that the eggs (Fig. 9-1b) are glued to the hairs of the head, especially over the ears and back of the head. Children, especially girls, have a higher incidence of head lice than adults. As the eggs are cemented to the bases of hairs, long hair *per se* is not more attractive than short hair, but people who neglect to wash and comb their hair encourage the build-up of lice. Strains of head lice that normally lay their eggs on straight hair, which is round in cross-section, often encounter difficulties in cementing their eggs at the base of the tightly coiled, oval-sectioned hair of negroid people. Thus, in a predominantly caucasian population, the incidence of head lice on the minority negroid people may be lower, while the converse may be true when negroid people outnumber non-negroids.

On average a person has only about 10–20 adult head lice, but occasionally larger infestations occur and may cause much scratching which can lead to scabs, secondary infections and pustules.

Head lice are spread by close contact, such as children playing together with their heads touching. There is very little evidence that lice are caught from hairdressers, backs of chairs or cinema seats.

9.1.3 *Pubic lice* (Pthirus pubis)

Pubic lice are slightly smaller (1.5–2.0 mm) than head or body lice but are distinctly broader, and the claws on the mid- and hind-legs are very large (Fig. 9-1d). Their shape and sluggish movements are responsible for the name crab lice.

Their life-cycle is similar to that of head lice, but the eggs are laid on hairs of the genital and perianal regions. Pubic lice are sometimes found on other coarse body hairs, such as those under the arms, on the chest, on beards and even on eyelashes! Eggs hatch within a week and the nymphal stage lasts about 10 days. Crab lice are usually caught through sexual intercourse. The French characteristically call them 'papillons d'amour'. Adults are more commonly infested than children, but if children sleep with infested adults then they will get lice. It is possible, although rare, to catch pubic lice from discarded underclothing and very unlikely to get them from lavatory seats – the two excuses most people give when seeking help to get rid of their pubic lice!

9.2 Medical importance

9.2.1 Nuisance

The presence of lice on people is referred to as pediculosis. All three species of lice can cause irritation and annoyance; by far the commonest are head lice. The repeated injection of saliva by large numbers of body lice during feeding, has a slight toxic affect that makes people feel depressed and irritable, in fact they feel 'lousy'.

9.2.2 Epidemic typhus

Epidemic typhus was very common in Ireland during the Potato Famine of 1845–47. The last big epidemic occurred in eastern Europe and Russia during 1917–23, when over 3 million people died; the Naples epidemic of 1943 was contained by killing the vectors with DDT. Typhus is now found sporadically in many countries, but especially in Africa.

Typhus is a rickettsial disease caused by *Rickettsia prowazeki* (named in honour of the American H.T. Ricketts and the Austrian von Prowazek, both of whom died experimenting with typhus). People with typhus develop fevers, headaches, a rash and become mentally confused. Adults are more severely affected than children; most untreated people over 50 years old die. A peculiar aspect of typhus is that after recovery the rickettsiae can persist in people at very low levels and be asymptomatic. However, when such persons are under stress, such as that caused by a family bereavement, recrudescences can occur. This phenomenon is known as Brill-Zinsser disease; the person becomes infective and if he has body lice, transmission can begin. Typhus can be successfully treated with good nursing and antibiotics.

All three louse species are capable of transmitting louse-borne typhus, but only body lice have been incriminated in typhus epidemics. Rickettsiae are ingested during feeding and enter the cells of the louse's stomach, and multiply there so enormously that after about 4 days they rupture the cells and rickettsiae are liberated into the lumen of the gut. Infection takes place when contaminated faeces are scratched into abrasions, come into contact with mucous membranes, or are inhaled. Rickettsiae remain infective in the louse's faeces for as long as 3 months. Vigorous scratching resulting in crushing lice can also lead to infection.

The rupturing of the stomach cells kills the louse after 8–10 days, making typhus a disease of the louse as well as of man. This partially explains why typhus patients often have few or no lice on their clothing, although their high temperatures also cause lice to abandon them.

9.2.3 Trench fever

Another disease spread by faeces of the body louse is trench fever or 5-day fever, caused by *Rochalimaea quintana*, which although painful is non-fatal and uncommon. As its name suggests it has been associated with troops living in trenches; it appeared in Europe in World War I (1914–18) and again during 1941–43 of World War II.

9.2.4   Louse-borne relapsing fever

Relapsing fevers are caused by spirochaetes, which are thin spiral organisms related to, but longer than, bacteria. One form is spread by body lice and is again associated with overcrowded living conditions and poor hygiene. Some of the more recent epidemics have been in Ethiopia. The causative organism is *Borrelia recurrentis.* (There are several other rather similar relapsing fevers caused by *Borrelia* species, but they are mostly spread by ticks.) After spirochaetes have been ingested with the louse's blood-meal they rapidly migrate across the stomach wall and enter the haemocoele and here they remain trapped. Transmission arises only when lice are crushed and the released spirochaetes enter scratches and abrasions or come into contact with mucous membranes. Clearly, squashing lice between the finger nails, or the practice in some communities of 'cracking' lice between the teeth, is to be avoided.

Patients suffering from relapsing fever develop symptoms rather like those caused by typhus. Relapsing fevers can be cured by a course of injections with penicillin or other suitable antibiotics given orally.

9.3   Control of lice

Shaving the head, or genital and perianal regions, is a drastic but effective method of combating head and pubic lice. Before the advent of efficient and safe insecticides, special steel combs with finely-set teeth were widely used to remove lice and nits from the head and even today, louse combs remain useful for removing unsightly nits that stay attached after insecticidal treatment.

Most body lice cling to clothing and are killed if clothes are washed in very hot water or subjected to dry heat of about 65–70°C for 30 minutes. The best procedure for ridding people of body lice is to apply insecticidal powders between the body and clothing. Dusting a person with 10% DDT can be very effective. This is a very safe formulation and there is no need for persons to remove their clothes or wash the DDT from their bodies.

Proprietry emulsions, lotions and creams containing benzyl benzoate or more commonly, insecticides like DDT, HCH, malathion or carbaryl, are widely used to kill head and pubic lice. A single treatment is sufficient unless DDT or HCH are used which do not kill the eggs, so necessitating another application 7–10 days later. Insecticidal preparations should remain on the head for 12–24 hours before the hair is washed, consequently insecticidal shampoos which are rinsed from the hair within minutes of application are not very effective.

The development of insecticide resistance by head and body lice in many areas is a problem, and requires the use of insecticides such as temephos (Abate), propoxur or pyrethrum.

10 Bedbugs

There are some 75 species of bedbugs, all belonging to the family Cimicidae of the order Hemiptera, but only two commonly feed on man, namely *Cimex lectularius* and *C. hemipterus*. The former has a more or less world-wide distribution, while *C. hemipterus* was originally confined to the tropics but has become increasingly common in temperate regions. The biology of both species is very similar and they look almost identical. Very occasionally, Cimicidae parasitic on other animals such as pigeons and bats, feed on people.

10.1 Biology of bedbugs

Bedbugs are flattish, wingless, brown, oval insects, 4–6 mm long (Fig. 10-1b). The head has a pair of small dark eyes, conspicuous 4-segmented antennae and a thin rigid proboscis closely appressed to the underside of the body, except during feeding when it is swung forwards. The prothorax has distinct wing-like expansions, while the meso- and metathorax are partially covered by small hemielytra. The abdomen is distinctly segmented, in males its tip is more pointed than in females and has a small curved penis. Female adults have a small V-shaped indentation on the left side of the ventral surface of the 4th abdominal segment, leading to a peculiar structure called the organ of Berlese or Ribaga. Since both sexes bite, distinguishing them is not important.

Bedbugs are relatively inactive during the day and hide away in mattresses, especially along their seams and in cracks and crevices in house structures and furniture. At night they become active and feed on sleeping occupants; very hungry bugs will also feed during the day. The yellowish-white eggs are covered with a delicate lattice-work pattern, are slightly but distinctly curved anteriorly, and have a small operculum (Fig. 10-1a). Female bedbugs may live for many months and lay several eggs a day which are cemented to rough surfaces or deposited in cracks and crevices in floorboards, furniture and other structures. They generally hatch in 8–11 days, but in hot countries hatching occurs in less than a week, while it may be delayed for several weeks in cold houses. The life-cycle is hemimetabolous and there are 5 nymphal stages each of which takes one or more blood-meals. Adults are formed after about 5–8 weeks, but this period can be prolonged for up to 6 months if it is cold or hosts are scarce. If bedbugs are unable to feed on man they may seek alternative hosts, such as rabbits, rats and other rodents, or even poultry and pigeons. In laboratory colonies, bedbugs have lived as long as 4 years and they can remain alive

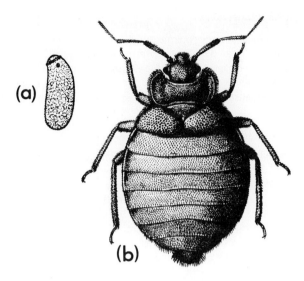

Fig. 10-1 Bedbugs (*Cimex lectularius*): (**a**) egg; (**b**) adult male bug. (From Smith, 1973, Courtesy of British Museum (Nat. Hist.), London.)

without food for 18 months.

The sexual act of bedbugs is unique in insects. The male's penis is not inserted into the female's genital opening, but is thrust through the cuticle on the left side of the 4th abdominal sternite. Spermatozoa are then injected into the organ of Berlese or Ribaga, which is really a copulatory pouch. After a few hours, spermatozoa pass from the pouch into the female's haemocoele and swim towards the bases of the oviducts, enter them and then migrate to the ovaries where fertilization ensues.

Because they are wingless, bedbugs have relatively poor powers of dispersal. Although they sometimes crawl from one house to another, the most important method of dissemination is through people's possessions such as furniture, mattresses, and more rarely clothes and baggage. Bedbugs are usually associated with poor quality houses and slums, but rehousing people in new premises does not always solve the problem, because people frequently carry their bugs with them in their belongings.

Bedbug-infested houses can be identified by unhatched and hatched eggs stuck to walls and in cracks of furniture, cast-off skins, living nymphs and adults hiding in cracks and crevices, and dark blood-spots on bed sheets. These spots are the bug's faeces, mostly composed of excess blood discharged during or shortly after, blood-feeding. Bedbugs have repugnatorial glands that emit a faint odour which can occasionally be detected in heavily infested houses, but usually such houses have much more powerful insanitary smells masking the bedbug's odour.

10.2 Medical importance

Bedbugs are thought not to transmit disease; they may possibly play a part in spreading viral hepatitis, but this needs clarification. In India, repeated feeding of large numbers of bedbugs on infants is reported to have caused iron deficiency. Although they are probably not vectors bedbugs can nevertheless cause much annoyance and many sleepless nights.

10.3 Bedbug control

Control consists of treating houses with insecticides. Liquid formulations of DDT, HCH, malathion and dichlorvos (DDVP) can be sprayed onto walls and furniture. Mattresses, (not those of infants) can also be lightly sprayed so long as they are dried afterwards; alternatively insecticidal dusts can be sprinkled on them. Addition of natural or synthetic pyrethrins to sprays is useful, as it irritates the bugs and flushes them out from their hiding places making them more exposed to insecticidal contact. Small insecticidal smoke cannisters are valuable for fumigating premises. In many parts of the world, bedbugs have unfortunately developed resistance to DDT, dieldrin, HCH and malathion, consequently, other insecticides have to be used.

11 Triatomine Bugs

The family Reduviidae contains many genera and species of superficially rather similar bugs, most of which are predacious on small arthropods, but about a hundred species, all belonging to the subfamily Triatominae, are blood-suckers. Most of them are found in South and Central America and southern parts of the USA, where they are known as cone-nose bugs, assassin bugs or kissing bugs. Several species, mainly of the genera *Triatoma*, *Rhodnius* and *Panstrongylus*, are vectors of *Trypanosoma cruzi* which causes Chagas' disease, also known as American trypanosomiasis. Some authorities consider that Charles Darwin contracted Chagas' disease during his voyage on HMS Beagle to South America.

11.1 Biology of triatomine bugs

Adults are large insects (1–4.5 cm) which are readily identified by their elongated snout-like heads which bear conspicuous 4-segmented antennae (Fig. 11-1b). As in bedbugs, the proboscis is appressed to the underside of the head except during feeding when it is swung forward. The pronotum is large and triangular, and combined with the long head is responsible for the name cone-nose bugs. The meso- and metathorax are hidden beneath the hemielytra which, like the membraneous hindwings, are fully functional. The segmented abdomen is hidden by the wings except for its margins. Many species are mainly brownish, but several have contrasting yellow, orange and red bands, mainly on the pronotum, the hard basal part of the hemielytra and around the edges of the abdominal segments. For the novice it is not easy to distinguish the sexes of triatomines, but this is not a serious disadvantage since both sexes suck blood.

The life-cycle is hemimetabolous and rather similar to that of bedbugs. The white or pinkish eggs have an unpatterned shell and a characteristic small constriction just before the operculum (Fig. 11-1a). They are usually glued into crevices of animal shelters such as rodent burrows and bird's nests, but also to walls, roofs and furniture of mud-walled and thatched-roofed village houses. Eggs normally hatch after 10–30 days, although in cool weather they may remain unhatched for up to 8 weeks. As in bedbugs, there are 5 nymphal stages, each one taking one or more blood-meals. At night, adults and nymphs will bite any exposed parts of sleeping people. When nights are cold and people are well wrapped, their faces may be the only accessible part – bites around the mouth have led to the name kissing bugs. Surprisingly for such large insects, bites are usually relatively painless. Young nymphs can ingest as much as 12 times their weight of

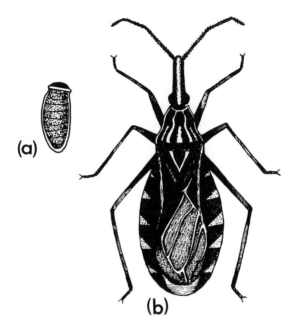

Fig. 11-1 Triatomine bug (*Rhodnius* species): (**a**) egg; (**b**) adult bug. (From Service, 1980.)

blood and as a consequence become inflated like red balloons; occasionally other nymphs and adults pierce their distended abdomens and obtain a 'second-hand' meal, without apparently harming the assaulted nymphs! Older nymphs and adults suck up only 3–4 times their weight in blood. Volumetrically, the biggest meals are taken by 5th-stage nymphs and can be as much as 600 mg. In heavily infested houses occupants can lose as much as 100 cm^3 blood a month! Sucking up such large quantities of blood may take 10–25 minutes, during which time the bugs often defaecate on their hosts, behaviour which has epidemiological implications (p. 69). Nymphal development takes a long time; even under optimum conditions it occupies 3–4 months, and more usually bugs remain as nymphs for about a year, while in some species the nymphal stage extends to 2 years. In the absence of suitable hosts, both nymphs and adults can survive 4–8 months of starvation.

The Triatominae are basically blood-feeders on wild animals inhabiting forests or semi-desert areas of Central and South America. Hosts include rodents, oppossums, armadillos, marsupials, bats, birds and iguanas. The bugs usually breed in their burrows or nests, or amongst foliage at the top of palm trees. A few species, however, have switched their attention to man, feeding and living in his houses, especially the rural dilapidated ones which are full of cracks and crevices. Infested houses can contain several thousand bugs. These bugs are opportunistic feeders, and apart from attacking man, they feed on cats, dogs, donkeys, cattle, goats, pigs and chickens, in fact, they are often very common in poultry sheds.

Although triatomines have well developed wings they do not fly far. Instead they crawl into nearby premises or get transported in furniture and baggage. They are also successful at hitch-hiking rides on buses and trains, as well as clinging to feathers of migratory birds.

11.2 Chagas' disease (*Trypanosoma cruzi*)

Chagas' disease (American trypanosomiasis) is present in all Central and South American countries. The causative agent, *Trypanosoma cruzi*, is initially in the blood but soon invades other tissues such as the heart muscles. This can cause a greatly enlarged heart, although this frequently does not happen for some years. The trypanosomes multiply in the muscles and other tissues and periodically reinvade the blood system. Chagas' disease is often regarded as a disease of middle-aged people because it is frequently asymptomatic in early life, then suddenly around 40 years heart failure occurs, especially after strenuous exercise. About 5-10% of people living in endemic areas are infected, but not all die or even show clinical symptoms. Unfortunately there is no really satisfactory drug for treating Chagas' disease, although some drugs can give 90% cure if given during the early stages of infection.

Infection can arise through eating food contaminated with the bug's faeces or inadequately cooked meat, such as the flesh of opossums having *T. cruzi*. While in turn, opossums can become infected through eating triatomine bugs. Occasionally the parasites cross the placenta and a baby is born infected. People may contract Chagas' disease through infected blood transfusions, but by far the commonest method of transmission is by triatomine bugs acting as vectors. Trypanosome parasites ingested with a blood-meal undergo multiplication in the insect's gut and after 1–2 weeks infective trypanosomes are present in the hindgut. Infection occurs when contaminated faeces, excreted while the bug is feeding, are scratched into abrasions or puncture wounds caused by the bug's bites, or get rubbed into the eyes or other mucous membranes.

Probably any triatomine species is capable of transmitting *T. cruzi*, but only those that have become domiciliated and readily feed on man are vectors (e.g. *Triatoma infestans*, *Rhodnius prolixus*, *Panstrongylus megistus*). Chagas' disease is a zoonosis, *T. cruzi* is principally a parasite of wild animals such as opossums, armadillos, urban rats and other rodents, carnivores and possibly bats. These animals, and also the bugs themselves, serve as reservoirs of infection for man. In a few areas, the parasites are restricted to animals, for instance *T. cruzi* is quite common in small mammals in Texas and California, but as the vectors do not bite man there are no human cases.

11.3   Control of triatomine bugs

Chagas' disease is a disease of the forgotten poor, not of the rich living in modern city houses, nor visitors sleeping in air-conditioned hotels.

As there are no effective prophylactic or curative drugs, control of Chagas' disease must be based on attacking the vectors. Theoretically, the solution is to rehouse people living in bug-infested hovels in new homes, made of cement blocks and corrugated metal roofs, which lack cracks and crevices in which the bugs can shelter. Provision of new homes, however, is costly and impractical except on a very limited scale. Consequently, vector control relies on spraying the interior of houses and various outbuildings (especially chicken sheds), with residual insecticides, particularly HCH and dieldrin. The former remains effective for about a month, whereas dieldrin persists for 2–3 months but is more toxic than HCH and so not so safe to use. Repetitive house-spraying as part of malaria campaigns has often provided the added bonus of reducing triatomine populations and the incidence of Chagas' disease. The problem with spraying houses, however, is that it kills only those bugs sheltering in them. It leaves untouched the large populations of bugs resting in natural shelters, which will readily invade houses after the insecticidal properties have worn off. Also, in some areas such as in Venezuela, vectors have developed resistance to HCH and dieldrin, but as yet this is not a major obstacle.

12 Other Blood-sucking Insects

The foregoing chapters have dealt with the important blood-sucking insects, but this book would be incomplete without reference, albeit briefly, to a few other haematophagous insects.

12.1 Stableflies

Stableflies, *Stomoxys calcitrans*, belong to the subfamily Stomoxinae of the Muscidae and have a worldwide distribution. Adults resemble houseflies (*Musca* spp.) and are often called biting houseflies, but are distinguished by having a rigid forwardly projecting proboscis. Both sexes take blood-meals from wild and domesticated animals and also from man. Biting occurs mainly out of doors during the day, and most bites are on the legs.

Eggs are laid in horse manure, compost pits and decaying vegetable matter, but rarely on human or animal faeces. They hatch within 1–3 days into creamy, typically maggot-shaped larvae. In hot weather, puparia are formed after about a week, but not until 4–5 weeks if temperatures are low; adults emerge after 1–3 weeks. In hot countries stableflies breed throughout the year, but in temperate regions they overwinter as adults in warm stables and outhouses, and feed intermittently through the winter.

Stableflies are most commonly encountered in rural areas, especially where there are horses, cattle or pigs. Because of their painful bites they can become a nuisance, but they are of no real medical importance, although they can occasionally be mechanical vectors of human and animal trypanosomiasis. They can also spread several protozoan and nematode parasites to wild and domestic animals.

Control consists of preventing the accumulation of manure and decomposing vegetable matter, or spraying it with insecticides. Residual insecticides applied to stables and cow sheds can help reduce breeding of stableflies.

12.2 Congo floor maggot

This peculiar insect is found only in tropical Africa (and Cape Verde Islands). Formerly called *Auchmeromyia luteola* it has recently been renamed *A. senegalensis*: together with blow-flies, it belongs to the family Calliphoridae. Adults are large flies (9–12 mm), dull yellow to brown, and have the 2nd abdominal segment about twice as long as any of the other 3 segments.

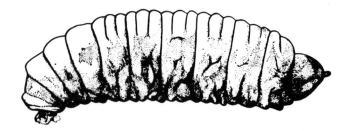

Fig. 12-1 Larva of Congo floor maggot (*Auchmeromyia senegalensis*). (From Smith, 1973, Courtesy of British Museum (Nat. Hist.) London.)

Eggs are deposited on the sandy floor of huts and hatch after 1–3 days. At night, larvae (Fig. 12-1) crawl towards people sleeping on the floor and take blood-meals from them. They feed once or twice a week, hiding in cracks and crevices during the day. A full grown larva measures 15 mm. Puparia are formed after about a month and adults, which do not suck blood, emerge about 11–14 days later. As larvae are unable to climb, people sleeping on beds raised on legs just a few centimetres high cannot be attacked. Previously this most unusual insect was quite common in certain parts of Africa, but it has now become much rarer.

12.3 Hornflies

These small flies all belong to the subfamily Stomoxinae of the family Muscidae. They resemble very small stableflies and are often known as hornflies because they bite round the bases of horns of cattle. All species belong to the genus *Haematobia* (e.g. *H. irritans*); formerly some were placed in the genera *Lyperosia* and *Siphona*.

12.4 Ectoparasitic flies

Three families of Diptera are ectoparasitic on mammals and birds and suck blood. These are the Nycteribiidae and Strebilidae, both of which are called bat flies because they feed exclusively on bats, and the Hippoboscidae (louse flies) which are ectoparasites of sheep, cattle, deer, goats and birds. These ectoparasitic flies are usually greatly flattened, have a leathery integument and are often wingless. They occasionally attack man.

12.5 Moths

A few moth species have the peculiar habit of settling on the face of cattle, wild mammals and sometimes man and feeding on eye discharges. One noctuid moth in Malaysia, *Calyptra eustrigata*, has gone a step further;

with its serrated proboscis, it penetrates the skin of rhinoceroses and elephants to suck up blood. So there is, in fact, a blood-sucking moth!

12.6 Acarines

This book is restricted to insects that suck blood, but it is appropriate to remind readers that other arthropods, such as ticks and some mites, are also haematophagous on man and a large variety of animals, and many are vectors of disease. For example, leptotrombiculid mites transmit scrub typhus in Asia and *Ornithodoros* ticks spread endemic relapsing fever in tropical and some temperate regions. Hard (ixodid) ticks are vectors in both tropical and temperate countries of numerous encephalitis viruses, and rickettsiae responsible for Rocky Mountain Spotted Fever, and other diseases. Ticks are also very important vectors of livestock diseases such as louping ill, a virus disease of sheep in Scotland and elsewhere in Europe, of Texas cattle fever and African East Coast fever of cattle.

Appendix

Some of the more common or important diseases transmitted to man and animals by blood-sucking insects.

Diseases	Pathogens	Vectors
Arboviruses		
African horse sickness	Virus	*Culicoides* midges
Bluetongue of sheep	Virus	*Culicoides* midges
Bovine ephemeral fever	Virus	*Culicoides* midges
Bunyamwere	Virus	Culicine mosquitoes
Chikungunya	Virus	Culicine mosquitoes
Dengue	Virus	Culicine mosquitoes
Encephalitis group (e.g. Japanese encephalitis, Eastern equine encephalitis)	Virus	Culicine mosquitoes
O'nyong nyong	Virus	Anopheline mosquitoes
Sandfly or papatacci fever	Virus	Phlebotomine sandflies
Yellow fever	Virus	Culicine mosquitoes
Rickettsiae		
Endemic (flea-borne) typhus	*Rickettsiae mooseri*	Fleas
Epidemic (louse-borne) typhus	*Rickettsiae prowazeki*	Body lice
Spirochaetes		
Louse-borne relapsing fever	*Borrelia recurrentis*	Body lice
Bacteria		
Bubonic plague	*Yersinia pestis*	Rat fleas
Tularaemia	*Francisella tularensis*	Horseflies

Bacteria-like

Bartonella fever or Carrion's disease	*Bartonella bacilliformis*	Phlebotomine sandflies

Protozoa

Chagas' disease or American trypanosomiasis	*Trypanosoma cruzi*	Triatomine bugs
Kala azar	*Leishmania donovani*	Phlebotomine sandflies
Leucozytozoon infections of birds	*Leucoytozoon* species	Blackflies
Malaria	*Plasmodium* species	Anopheline mosquitoes
Nagana or animal trypanosomiasis	*Trypanosoma* species	Tsetse flies
Oriental sore	*Leishmania tropica*	Plebotomine sandflies
Sleeping sickness or human trypanosomiasis	*Trypanosoma gambiense* and *T. rhodesiense*	Tsetse flies

Filarial nematode worms

Bancroftian filariasis	*Wuchereria bancrofti*	Anopheline and culicine mosquitoes
Brugian filariasis	*Brugia malayi*	Culicine mosquitoes
Dog heartworm	*Dirofilaria immitis*	Culicine mosquitoes
Loiasis	*Loa loa*	*Chrysops* flies
Onchocerciasis or river blindness	*Onchocerca volvulus*	Blackflies
"Mansonelliasis"	*Mansonella* species	Blackflies and *Culicoides* midges

Cestode worms

Dog tapeworm	*Dipylidium caninum*	Fleas

Further Reading

ANDREWS, M.L.A. (1976). *The Life that Lives on Man.* Faber and Faber, London.

BAKER, J.R. (1982). *The Biology of Parasitic Protozoa.* Studies in Biology No. **138**. Edward Arnold, London.

BATES, M. (1949). *The Natural History of Mosquitoes.* Macmillan, New York, republished by Harper Torchbooks (1965).

BRUCE-CHWATT, L.J. and DE ZULUETA, J. (1980). *The Rise and Fall of Malaria in Europe. A Historico-epidemiological Study.* Oxford University Press, Oxford.

BUSVINE, J.R. (1976).*Insects, Hygiene and History.* The Athlone Press, London.

BUSVINE, J.R. (1980). *Insects and Hygiene. The Biology and Control of Insects Pests of Medical and Domestic Importance.* Chapman and Hall, London.

CLOUDSLEY-THOMPSON, J.L. (1976). *Insects and History.* Weidenfeld and Nicolson, London.

GILLETT, J.D. (1971). *Mosquitos.* Weidenfeld and Nicolson, London.

HARRISON, G. (1978). *Mosquitoes, Malaria and Men: A History of the Hostilities Since 1880.* Macmillan, London.

HARWOOD, R.F. and JAMES, M.T. (1979). *Entomology in Human and Animal Health.* Macmillan, New York.

KETTLE, D.S. (1984). *Medical and Veterinary Entomology.* Croom Helm, London.

LAIRD, M. (ed) (1977). *Tsetse: The Future for Biological Methods in Integrated Control.* International Development Research Centre, Ottawa.

LAIRD, M. (ed) (1981). *Blackflies. The Future for Biological Methods in Integrated Control.* Academic Press, London.

MANSON-BAHR, P.E.C. and APTED, F.I.C. (1982). *Manson's Tropical Diseases.* Ballière Tindall, London.

MARSHALL, A.G. (1981). *The Ecology of Ectoparasitic Insects.* Academic Press, London.

MATTINGLY, P.F. (1969). *The Biology of Mosquito-borne Disease.* George Allen and Unwin, London.

MUIRHEAD-THOMSON, R.C. (1968). *Ecology of Insect Vector Populations.* Academic Press, London.

MUIRHEAD-THOMSON, R.C. (1982). *Behaviour Patterns of Blood-sucking Flies.* Pergamon, Oxford.

NASH, T.A.M. (1969). *Africa's Bane; The Tsetse Fly.* Collins, London.

PHILLIPS, R.S. (1983). *Malaria*. Studies in Biology No. **152**. Edward Arnold, London.

SERVICE, M.W. (1980). *A Guide to Medical Entomology*. Macmillan, London.

SERVICE, M.W. (1981). Ecological considerations in biocontrol strategies against mosquitoes. *Biocontrol of Medical and Veterinary Pests*, M. Laird (ed), pp. 193–195. Praeger, New York.

SHOLDT, L.L., HOLLOWAY, M.L. and FRONK, W.D. (1979). *The Epidemiology of Human Pediculosis in Ethiopia*. Special publication of Naval Air Station, Jacksonville, Florida, USA.

SMITH, K.G.V. (ed) (1973). *Insects and other Arthropods of Medical Importance*. British Museum (Natural History), London.

WILLMOTT, S. (ed) (1978). *Medical Entomology Centenary*. Symposium Proceedings of the Royal Society of Tropical Medicine and Hygiene, London.

Index